Not So Fast

Not So Fast

by Sarah McMahon

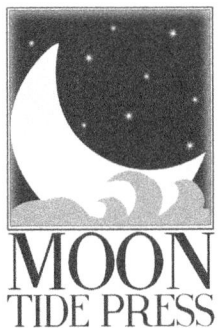

~ 2026 ~

Not So Fast
© Copyright 2026 Sarah McMahon
All rights reserved. No part of this book may be used or reproduced in any manner whatsoever without written permission from either the author or the publisher, except in the case of credited epigraphs or brief quotations embedded in articles or reviews.

Editor-in-chief
Eric Morago

Operations Associate
Shelly Holder

Associate Editors
Katrina Prow
Mackensi E. Green
Allysa Murray
Ellen Webre

Editor Emeritus
Michael Miller

Cover design
Andrea Smith

Book design
Michael Wada

Moon Tide logo design
Abraham Gomez

Not So Fast
is published by Moon Tide Press

Moon Tide Press
6709 Washington Ave. #9297
Whittier, CA 90608
www.moontidepress.com

FIRST EDITION

Printed in the United States of America

ISBN # 978-1-957799-46-9

CONTENTS

Prologue	6
Home	9
High School Dirtbags	13
Butch	18
California Redneck	22
Cancer's Best Friend is Cancer	27
The Big A (Anorexia)	32
Moving Day	36
IOU	43
Dr. Brille de Ramirez	48
You Are Going to Learn So Much	52
Help, I Broke My Hip	54
Work Sucks	59
Rock Bottom	69
Let's Talk About Menstruation	78
The Adults in the Room	82
Hey, Coach	86
Bad Boyfriend	91
Yes, You Can	102
Guns & Stuff	104
Dr. T. and Amy the Dietitian	108
Vegan No More	114
Waiting Room 2	118
Intuitive Eating	122
What Doesn't Make You Stronger	127
Returning	129
Anxious-Avoidant Attachment	137
Sad, Beautiful Women	142
Bad Dates	149
Mike Mike	156
Irritating Fudge	159
White Christmas	163
In the Short Term	167
Seasonally Depressive	170
Home Again	174
The End	178
About the Author	*180*
Acknowledgements	*181*

PROLOGUE

I am not a terrifically smart person. Luckily, being terrifically smart is increasingly rare, and if the state of our world is any indication, average intelligence is plummeting fast. If you're reading this book, know that you're smarter than the 44 percent of Americans who will not bother to pick up a book this year.

My name is Sarah, wife of Abraham and Mother of Isaac. Just kidding, I'm not biblical and I'm also not yet married. My only child is a 16-year-old orange dumpster cat. I was born in 1993, when *Sarah* was the third most popular baby name for girls in the good 'ole US of A. My middle name is Rose, and if you're thinking "*Rose*, what a pretty name," then you and my mother have a lot in common. When I asked my mother *why* she named me Sarah Rose, she said, "I just liked how it sounded." I did not dig deeper, because my family understands that some parts of life contain no mystery. My mother never had the time or energy to beat around the bush, indulge in astronomy, or wonder why names were names. She and my father are salt-of-the earth Midwestern people who laugh at a good fart joke and pray before dinner. My father is not a boisterous man and has never seen the sense in celebrating himself. Last Father's Day I called to tell him "*Happy Father's Day*" and he just said, "Oh. Huh."

Our last name is McMahon, and that's the part of our name that gets a bit sticky. My grandmother gave birth to my father when she was only seventeen and did what most gals in the 1960's did when they found themselves pregnant too early or out of wedlock; she married the guy. His name was Arthur and for reasons unknown to me, he didn't hang around long. My grandmother went on to endure four subsequent marriages, her second and third to the same man, Larry McMahon. Larry legally adopted my father, so I now share a last name with a nice family in Florida whom I have never met and who will likely never read this book. I've only ever been to Florida once, but when I was there, I ran into an alligator on the side of a road and figured I'd seen enough of the sunshine state. Every now and then, when I introduce myself to people over a certain age, they'll say, "Any relation to Ed McMahon?" and I'll wink and say, "I wish!" I bear no blood relation to any of the most famous McMahon's, and most certainly not Linda.

Once, when I was visiting the Hollywood Walk of fame, a round man in suspenders and wide black glasses stopped me on the sidewalk, "one of these stars down here for you?" he asked, gesturing at the ground. I stared at him the way you might stare at an asteroid before answering, "Oh no, I'm not famous. But Ed McMahon was my great grandfather!" and walked away shimmying my hips before he could reply. Visiting L.A. was fun, if a bit exhausting, like going to a museum where the statues demanded to talk to you. I figured it didn't matter what I said, since I would never see him again.

I am not a native Californian, but I do live here now, in a leaky apartment near the coast in Orange County. I grew up on a farm outside a nondescript town in Northwestern Wisconsin called Colfax. Our biggest claim to fame was that the town sits halfway between the Equator and the North pole. There's a sign downtown by the river that says so. Sometimes in the spring, when the water in that river was high, kids would jump into it from an imposing bridge. I never did that, because I like living.

There are roughly 1,200 residents of Colfax, and when I graduated from high school in 2011, there were only 60 students in my graduating class. Not to toot my own horn or anything, but I was good at memorizing facts and therefore graduated at the top of my very small class. I had to give a commencement speech, and I wrote it in the form of a Dr. Seuss style poem: "A is for awesome, because that's what we are, B is for brilliant and bound to go far," etc. It's only embarrassing if you say it out loud.

Colfax has no stop lights and only a handful of stop signs. There is a small grocery store on one side of town, where produce is grossly overpriced, but beer is cheap. There is a Dollar General, two gas stations, a bowling alley, and some antique shops that are only open once a week. An establishment downtown called the Bucksnort Bar displays a statue of a deer lying on its back guzzling a beer. My hometown is not classy and the people who reside there enjoy quiet, space, gas station coffee, and driving slowly. There is no point in rushing, because there is nowhere to go and nothing in the way of getting there.

Colfax is the sort of town where kids drive snowmobiles to school and skip class to go deer hunting. It is quintessential Toby Keith Americana, complete with a heavy dose of flags, pickup trucks, and modest white-sided housing. We shopped at Kohls, Shopko, and thrift stores. We stoked a lot of campfires, raised a lot of cattle, and drank too much, far too young. My hometown was quaint and safe and unable to contain my yearning for adventure. I preferred running through the forest or walking barefoot through the thick mud of our vegetable garden to wearing dresses, doing makeup, or talking about boys. In fact, I still don't see the point in talking about boys. When women talk about men, all they're really talking about is how they'd like to be loved, or how they haven't been, or how they should be.

This isn't a book about a small town though. It's a book about growing up, rural America, and starting over. It's a book about running and eating disorders and broken relationships. It's a book about my life, and I think that's interesting because I'm me. The stereotype of memoirs is that you have to be famous to write one. I am happily not famous, so I know that, prior to picking up this book, you have never heard of me. I want you to know that I'm grateful you're here, and I'm insanely happy you've chosen to read my story.

HOME

My father sat at our oval Formica-topped kitchen table, on a chipped wooden chair that has been in that kitchen, around that table, since my great-grandparents built the house in 1950-something. My father has a dark beard and not much hair. He wears wire rimmed glasses and a t-shirt I gave him last Christmas, from the infamous Los Rios Street in San Juan Capistrano, CA. The kitchen he sits in is over a thousand miles away from Los Rios Street, in a house situated on a small hillside in rural Northwest Wisconsin.

"Hey!" he says, smirking, "tell Mike there's a house they call the rising sun," before chuckling to himself, a toothpick bouncing up and down from his laughing mouth. "The Animals!" he cries, gesticulating with his hands, "I can't believe you didn't know that!"

House of the Rising Sun is my ringtone and has been for as long as I can remember. Whenever my then-boyfriend calls, my father yells, "Tell Mike there's a house! They call the rising sun!" One night, he will demand that I sit on the brown sofa in the living room as he streams the original music video, released the year he was born, to the large, flat screen television. The Animals wear matching yellow suits and play the song while gazing into the camera, *and it's been the ruin of many a poor boy and God I know I'm one.*

I live in Southern California (hence the t-shirt from Los Rios Street), but I grew up here, in the house my parents still live in. Rural Wisconsin is worlds away from Southern California, and I've made it my personal mission to distinguish how. It's the same country, after all. We speak the same language. Or do we?

My father blows his nose, and it sounds like one of the freight trains that roll through town every day. "Drier than a day-old popcorn fart in here," he mutters, before heading downstairs to check the humidifier. The basement is half finished with orange carpet. There is a rarely used pool table down there too, with the canonical picture of dogs on hind legs, teeing up a perfect shot. One winter when I was young, we sat in this basement for hours shucking hundreds of cobs of popcorn. Like many of my father's ventures, the summer of popcorn started as an idea and ended with us being way in over our heads. The heavy metal handheld tool we used for shucking left my small hands red and raw, but the bowls of perfect yellow kernels made the slow work that much more satisfying. We ate that popcorn for years.

My father delighted in showing me the original *House of the Rising Sun* video, in part because he could. What I mean is, my parents gained access to high-speed internet in 2021, the result of a nationwide effort to bring internet access to more rural communities. Prior to this effort, my parents could not stream a video, making Netflix, Hulu, HBO, even YouTube all irrelevant. They had about 20 channels to choose from, ranging from the major networks (ABC, NBC, FOX) to hyper-local Wisconsin PBS programming. My mother likes to give money during the PBS annual appeals, and there are mugs in the cupboard to prove it.

My father's grandparents built the house my parents now own and farmed the land my parents purchased from them for $500 an acre. The land is part cornfield my parents rent out to a local farmer, woods where my brother and father hunt deer, and a large swamp with a creek running through it. My father has a way of ruminating on things, and has told me countless times how he'd like his body handled, whenever God decides to call him home.

"Have me burned," he says, "and toss my ashes in the creek in the springtime, when the water is high." His funeral, he insists, should not be a sad affair. "Have a party in the barn," he says with total seriousness, "like the Hank Williams Jr. song. I'll leave a list of music, but I want it to be a *party*."

The list includes songs like "Boondocks," "A Country Boy Can Survive," "God's Country," and "Copperhead Road." My father's mother (and my only surviving grandmother) hates when he talks about dying.

"If they toss you in the creek there won't be a stone to remember you by!" she protests. "Ma, I'll be *dead*," my father intones, grumbling to himself, "can't even have a say in how I die."

My mother, God bless her, stands by patiently waiting and listening, rolling her eyes. No one notices.

My father has lived well over half of his life on this farm, in the house on the small hill, sitting around the same Formica-topped table on those scuffed up wooden chairs. He wants to be dumped in the creek because this place; the house, the garden, the forest, the farm, the large wooden table, are home.

My father has a habit of repeating jokes, and his *House of the Rising Sun* joke landed no less than seven times. When I was in grade school, I went to a birthday party and came home with a puppy, a fuzzy golden mutt we named Chloe. Chloe had an idyllic life, but her one downfall was that she was allergic to corn. In the autumn when the corn was high and tasseling, she would run into the garden or cornfield to snag a cob or two. Then, she would spend the next 48 hours gnawing her feet, saliva dripping down her face as she bit and scratched, her eyes crossing madly. The vet prescribed a steroid, and one of its side effects was weight gain. So, every autumn, Chloe would go on steroids, gain a good ten pounds, and my father would walk around crowing, "Chloe's on the 'roids again!"

On summer nights, long before the internet was anywhere close to high speed, my parents, my brother, and I gathered in the living room to watch the nightly news, the gentle intonations of local newscasters lulling me to sleep. Tree frogs sang in the swamp and the air hung heavy with dew. Sometimes on clear nights, we would gather outside, gazing up at a blanket of stars. My mother would look up in wonder, every time. "There's no way this all happened by accident," she'd say.

And the days melted together, time stood still and simultaneously sprinted with breakneck speed. I went away to college, landed my first job in Chicago, and eventually moved to California.

Sometimes I call home at dinnertime, when my parents are sitting down at that Formica table, on those scuffed wooden chairs.
"Why don't you call me back when you're done?" I say. Sometimes they do, and sometimes they set the phone on the table in between them and say, "It's okay honey. We can talk."

HIGH SCHOOL DIRTBAGS

"Sarrrah," my teacher droned, not looking up from his attendance sheet. I was sitting in my 10th grade, third period history class, which I disliked because it always seemed to drag on unnecessarily long. To pass the time, I doodled in the margins of my planner, filling page after page in heavy black ink.

I numbly chirped, "Here," and continued staring out the window. I was wearing jeans and my boyfriend's hooded sweatshirt, which was two sizes too big and hung halfway down my thin thighs. My boyfriend went to a different school, nearly an hour's drive away, so I was only able to see him on weekends. I enjoyed the space between us, as well as the social capital that having a boyfriend granted me. As a 17-year-old girl, the hallmark of being cool was wearing an oversized sweatshirt that smelled of Axe body spray and teenage-boy sweat.

I was in my third period history class, and I was exhausted. I was up at 5:00 a.m. to run on my treadmill in the basement before showering, making breakfast, and driving to school with my brother, who was only a year ahead of me. The landscape outside was bleak and colorless, the bare trees reaching towards heaven as if begging God to rescue them from their cold misery. The temperature had not risen above ten degrees for a week, and the snow outside was icy and pocketed with dirt. I disliked winter and I disliked sitting in class and I even disliked going to basketball practice after school, even though there was nothing else for me to do.

My teacher, like a lot of teachers toward the end of their career, was simply waiting to retire. Rumor had it that, when he was a new teacher fresh out of college, he married one of his students. He was a bit charming and a bit aloof, which made him one of my favorites. At the beginning of the year, when my teacher handed out our books, I noticed that the first name written on the inside of the front cover was dated *1980*. The book was nearly 30 years old and falling apart. *Why are our books so old?* I thought. Our books looked like I felt; ragged and worn and tired. I was so, so, *tired*, and I had two more classes until lunch, when I'd eat a baggie of carrot sticks and a slice of bread with peanut butter on it. Sometimes, I'd stare at friends' lunches and fantasize about eating their food. Sometimes, the lunch ladies would give me another half of a peanut butter sandwich, which they always kept on hand for the kids who didn't like whatever MRE-adjacent food was on the menu.

In high school, my life was punctuated by food, my need for more but desire for less. I was a three-sport athlete, constantly on the move, and never eating enough for my level of activity. I liked the dead feeling in my legs as I sat in hard, uncomfortable classroom chairs. I liked doing something that I knew none of my peers were doing; running a bunch and slowly, deliberately starving myself thin. I craved the feeling of invincibility I gained by exercising my willpower and embracing my manic desire to succeed at something.

People who don't know much about eating disorders think that the media is the root cause of them, and certainly, the media doesn't help. But I grew up on a farm with limited interaction with the outside world and very limited access to media. We only had a few TV channels and barely had internet. My media came largely in the form of print–books, magazines, newspapers, and advertisements. I'd read the backs of cereal boxes, my grandmothers' old copies of *Reader's Digest*, and musty books I found in our basement. I grew up in the early 2000s when skinny jeans were popular and celebrities bigger than a size two were plastered on the covers of magazines. I vividly remember when Jessica Simpson, at the time a size six, became the subject of cruel bullying and body shaming. Even though I didn't have immediate access to media, the media I did have glorified thinness in what I've later come to realize is a tale as old as time.

Despite whatever role the media played in making me self-conscious, the most damning interactions occurred in real life. I was in fourth grade when a boy at school called me fat, which is exactly when I became acutely aware of my body. He was a standard bully, with the standard bully timeline: Popular-Bully-Kid picks on everyone and thereby earns social status. But Popular-Bully-Kid has few real friends because everyone is low-key afriad of him. He remained a popular-bully throughout our schooling, all the way until graduation. Now, popular-bully-kid is a slightly-overweight, mediocrely attractive father living on the outskirts of the small, Midwestern town I grew up in.

I couldn't see the future at the time though, all I could see was that popular-bully-kid made my life at school a living nightmare and I barely knew him. He bullied me so ruthlessly that nobody at school wanted to be seen with me, so I learned how to be alone. I spent recess reading books or playing touch football with a group of boys who didn't seem to care that I was a social outcast. They weren't really my friends, but they were impressed that I could run fast, and it became a point of pride that I was able to keep up with them. After school, I climbed onto a tattered school bus, looking forward to escaping into the woods behind my parents' house, where I played alone and felt the tenseness I held all day at school slowly evaporate.

Because Popular-Bully-Kid made fun of me for being fat, I started writing little workout plans for myself, not because I enjoyed the process of working out so much as I knew that working out (coupled with starving) was the best way to not become fat. Or at least, that's what I read in newspapers and magazines. So, I started not eating sweets, and later my restriction extended further, to any number of foods I deemed "unhealthy," like bread, potatoes, cereal, dried fruit, butter, eggs, and anything wrapped in packaging. In sixth grade, I joined the cross-country team, and then, I started winning races. Popular-Bully-Kid stopped picking on me as my name appeared in newspaper headlines.

My obsession with exercise and my dedication to winning was fueled by a need to prove to the world, and to myself, that I was good enough, that I was mentally tough, capable, and above all, *not fat.*

As a runner, I also internalized the belief that I needed to stay the same size forever or else lose my speed. Dozens of voices perpetuated this belief. My history teacher, for one, announced in front of my class after my most winning season, that I needed to be careful, because girls tend to slow down as they hit puberty. Later, the college coaches who recruited me echoed this sentiment and I latched onto their words as if they were the gospel truth. I learned that growing into a woman meant I'd be slower and less of an athlete, which is a pretty egregious lie, but I believed it nonetheless.

Back in my history classroom, my teacher snapped me out of a daze, "Sarah," he said again, more sharply this time, and I looked up from my planner, "You've been called to the office," he said, "you'd better go."

I was called to the office a lot back then, usually to pick up recruiting letters and packages from colleges, and that day was no different, a fat package of marketing materials from St. Norbert's college in De Pere, Wisconsin. When I first started receiving letters, I loved being called to the office because it made me feel special. I was getting attention from important people in places that were not my hometown. I was wanted. I mattered.
Soon, the thrill of being called to the office was replaced by tedium and eventually, scorn from some of my peers. One of my classmates was especially annoyed, and let it be known. She was a different kind of bully than popular-bully-kid, because she was a girl, and mean girls are nothing like mean boys. Mean boys call you fat and make fun of you to your face. Mean girls make fun of your clothes, your body, your personality, and your brain behind your back as they compliment your style, your demeanor, your grades. Mean girls act like your friend while they unravel your reputation with deliberate precision.

Mean Girl wasn't that good at hiding her meanness, though. When she smiled at me, she reminded me of Ursula from the Little Mermaid, her mouth too wide and too eager, like she was a cat, and I was a mouse. The way I overcame Popular-Bully-Kid was to prove him wrong. I was winning races. I was a good athlete. I was successfully delaying puberty. I was not fat. Important people were recruiting me from all over the country. I had tangible proof that he was wrong, so he moved on. The way I overcame Mean Girl was to simply ignore her. At the time, I wasn't fully aware that my indifference was ultimately what defeated her pleasure in tormenting me. I was simply too tired to care. And, since Popular-Bully-Kid had already tormented me and positioned me as a social outcast, I was used to being alone. Nothing Mean Girl did or said could change the fact that I'd learned to depend on myself. Instead, I found kinship with the nerds and misfits, the kids who felt isolated and outcast just like I did.

My best friend from high school is witty and quirky and so smart she carved a path from her home on a rural dead-end street straight to the doors of Princeton. Our public school did the best it could, but it did not, *could* not, prepare her or I for the rigors of higher education. Both of us felt punched in the face once we got to college, her by the Ivy League coursework and me by the fierce athletic competition. We were two large fish in a small pond who had to figure out the hard way that fish often grow as big as their environment will let them.

Fast forward more than a decade and she is studying for her law degree while I am at a tradeshow, selling a software platform for special events.

My birthday is tomorrow, so she sends me a text that reads: *"Happy Birthday's Eve."*

Thank you! I replied, *I'm at a trade show, yeehaw.*

'I'm at a tradeshow' is the most 30-year-old sentence I've ever heard, she replied.

Then, on my actual birthday, she wrote: *"Grateful to have you as a friend these last 15+ years. Also, that is such a long time. Our friendship has its learner's permit."*

BUTCH

"Why was she talking to you about me?" my grandmother demanded. We were outside in her gardens, where we spent most of our time during the long, humid midwestern summers. The "she" she was referring to was her own mother, my great-grandmother Irene Maves. Irene lived in a blue double-wide next to my parent's farmhouse. Irene and her late husband, Wilmer, built the house I grew up in and sold it to my parents with the contingency that they live out their remaining days in a trailer home on the farm.

I was barely ten years old, and my curiosity about my family grew as I grew able to understand the intricacies of what the adults talked about. From their conversations, I understood that my grandmother had been married not once, not twice, but five times to four different men. As a little girl, I could hardly imagine getting married once.

"Why did grandma get married so many times?" I'd asked Irene the previous afternoon. My great-grandmother was a frank woman with poor eyesight and even poorer hearing. She was tall, Norwegian, with specific ideas about how life should be lived and a soft spot for children and cats.

"You'd have to ask her honey," she told me, "I can't say I really understand myself, but I will say it was a bit too much."

With the unselfconscious energy of a ten-year-old, I decided I'd do just what Irene suggested and ask my grandmother myself. "Grandma," I said, as I squatted deeply to reach a stubborn weed tucked beneath a hosta plant, "why did you get married five times?"

"Who told you I got married five times?" she asked, pausing with a trowel in her hand to look hard at me.
"Great grandma," I answered, "she said *it was all a bit too much.*"

"Why was she talking to you about me?" she demanded, "it's none of her business and none of yours," her tone was sharp, and I understood that the conversation was over. I also understood that my grandmother's anger was more complicated than it seemed. There was something else in her voice that I couldn't recognize. Maybe it was disdain. Maybe it was fear. Either way, I did not know my paternal grandfather, and never would.

My inquisitiveness about my paternal grandfather grew as I transitioned from a rambunctious teenager into a young adult. My curiosity was influenced in part by my desire to know my family, and in part to understand how families can so easily fracture. After visiting my doctor for an annual checkup and keeping the "family history" section of the intake form necessarily vague, I decided to find my grandfather. It was not hard to track him down, and I discovered that he lived less than twenty miles from the farm where I grew up. I was twenty-six by then and already in California, a mostly-functional adult with too many bills and too much time on my hands.

The phone rang twice before he picked up, "Hello?" His voice sounded like the voice of any other old man. It was gentle but scratchy, like he had dryer lint stuck in his throat.

"My name is Sarah," I said, "You don't know me, but I think you know my dad."

"Ohh yes. Sarah," he said, pausing. "I did know your father." The past tense was not lost on me. "I know who you are," he continued. That last admission came as a surprise. I thought *I'd* found *him*, but he had known about me for a very long time.

"Have you talked to him, ever?" I ask.

After a pregnant pause, he answered, "No. I don't know what to tell you. That was a long time ago. We were kids. And I guess we decided to give it up." Give up *what*, I wasn't sure.

"I watched you in the papers," he said, "you were an amazing runner. You caused quite a stir here in Colfax." Against my will, tears pierced my eyes. He knew my name. Of course, he did. He'd read about me in the local newspaper, but he likely hadn't heard anything in years.

"Do you live around here? Are you married?"

"No," I answered, "I live in California. I was engaged, but we broke it off."

"Sometimes stuff like that just doesn't work out," he mused. "California. Wow. Do you ever get back up here?"

"I do, always for Christmas and usually once in the summer. It's so much nicer to visit in August," I quipped, a lame attempt to lighten the air between us.

"Well, I'd love to see you when you come back," my grandfather told me. "Why don't you give me a call this Christmas? It's so good to hear from you."

"I will," I told him, knowing I wouldn't.

I'm not sure what I wanted. Answers, maybe, so that I could easily justify his absence and his puzzling closeness. But like so many things, Arthur was not easily labeled. He had reasons, and there were circumstances I would never understand. As I dialed his number, I was expecting and half-wanting him hang up, to remain as silent as he'd been for most of my life. What I wasn't expecting to hear in his voice was kindness. I wasn't expecting to hear longing. And I certainly wasn't expecting to hear joy.

I never called Arthur when I went home that Christmas. Part of me didn't want to, and part of me was afraid of what might happen, and what my family might think. Only months after I neglected to call him, Arthur died at the age of 78, his wife and golden retriever by his side. His obituary was short and to the point. Arthur's friends and family called him Butch. He never had more children. He was married to his second wife for 42 years. He had four golden retrievers, all named Poncho. He liked to fish and was a good dancer. His obituary ended with, "God chooses the best and Butch is one of them."

My family rarely talked about Arthur, other than to insinuate his lack of character. My grandmother told me that he was not a good person, but I can't help but wonder how bad he really was. After all, I am a piece of him, whether I like it or not. He is just as inextricable from me as anyone else in my family. There is no good way to make peace with someone who is gone, no good way to connect dots that are only growing more faint with time. I wished I had more answers, a neat, bulleted list like teachers handed out in grade school. Here are the questions, and here is a key, neatly labeled and color coordinated. But life doesn't hand out answer sheets, it just keeps rolling forward, leaving us all to rectify the wrinkles in our hearts and smooth them out as best we can.

CALIFORNIA REDNECK

My great-grandmother Irene was one of my favorite people. She was 78 by the time I was born, and she always had time for me. Plus, she let me get away with things that most other people wouldn't, like playing with the sagging flesh of her upper arms. "Your arms will be like this too, someday," she'd laugh, before shuffling a deck of cards for another game of rummy. She had a mug in one of her cupboards with a Swedish table prayer printed in English on one side, and in Swedish on the other. Sometimes, at my pleading, she'd pull it out of the cupboard and read it to me: *"I Jesu navn / gar vi til bords / a spise og drikke / pa ditt ord / deg gud til aere, oss til gavn / sa far vi mat / I Jesu navn"*

> *In Jesus' name*
> *to the table we go*
> *to eat and drink*
> *according to his word*
> *to God the honor, us the gain*
> *so we have food*
> *in Jesus' name*

Irene read her bible each morning and ate prunes on shredded wheat. She kept a big Tupperware container of cookies in one of her cupboards, low enough for small hands to reach. There was an old book of fairy tales, the *real* kind, on her bottom bookshelf that she would read to me when I was sick. She kept photo albums beneath her TV filled with pictures of extended family; my father when he was young, my grandmother, my great-aunts and uncles and too many cousins to count. Sometimes I'd pick flowers from one of our wild, sprawling gardens and leave them on her doorstep. Sometimes I'd pick dandelions, and she would keep those, too. I loved visiting her house, but most of all, I loved how much she loved me.

"*Iiiissshhh*," Irene grumbled as she tried to thread a needle. It was summertime, and my brother and I were home all day while my parents worked. We spent a lot of time with my great grandmother after all our chores were done, hanging laundry on the line, picking green beans, mowing the lawn, raking the leaves and sticks that cluttered the yard after a thunderstorm. The summer heat came in undulating waves, and on the longest, hottest summer days we sat around the kitchen table, beneath a plastic golden chandelier, and played cards to pass the time.

"Let me help you," I said, taking the needle and thread in my small hands and cutting the end of the thread so it was no longer frayed. In a few seconds, the needle was threaded, and Irene smiled. "Thank you honey," she said, "It's so hard for me to see."

A few years later, I was in middle school. Every afternoon, the bus dropped me off at the end of her driveway and I'd skip up the stairs, fling open her door and shut it quietly behind me. Irene napped most afternoons, her black and white cat curled up next to her on a patchwork quilt that covered her full-sized bed. Above the bed were black and white photos of her three daughters, and a larger one of her and Wilmar, before age sucked the glow from their cheeks. Every day, I'd wake her up from her nap and we'd chat a bit before I'd head outside to take the dog for a walk in the woods behind the farmhouse.
One day, she blinked up at me. "Honey," she said, "if one day, you come in here and I don't wake up, you know what to do?"

I didn't want to say, because saying *yes* would mean acknowledging that one day, she wouldn't be there anymore. I knew about death, because one of our dogs had passed away–a German Shepard named Sheba, who had one floppy ear and one that pointed straight up. I knew that death was real, and I also knew to call my mother, or 911, if anything terrible happened.

"You call 911, okay?" she took my hand, her skin thin and translucent, age spotted and blue-veined. I gave her a small smile, hoping to reassure her that I was capable in times of crisis. I didn't know that I was, yet. That was something I'd learn much later.

"Okay Grandma," I said, secretly hoping, as most kids do, that everyone I loved would live forever. Nobody would need to call 911.

A few years later, shortly before I turned 15, Irene suffered a stroke. She recovered fine, and moved into a nursing home in town, just down the street from my high school. Her house sat empty, a dark gaping hole in the landscape of home. Irene liked the nursing home, the activities they planned, how she didn't have to cook, how there were other people around all day for her to talk to. Only a few short weeks after she was admitted to the nursing home, she suffered another stroke. This time, however, she did not recover, and she never woke up. She lay unconscious for days before she slipped into the next life, leaving a hole in my heart a thousand miles wide.

My father came into my bedroom the night she passed away. "Grandma's gone, sweetie," he said, gently rubbing my back. From my bedroom window, I could see her trailer house, the lights that usually glowed each night, where she sat at the kitchen table reading her Bible or playing solitaire. My father was crying, and I'd never seen him cry before. "Do you want to sit up for a bit?" he asked. But I just rolled over, facing the window where my grandmother no longer was, holding on tight to my heartache.

I held onto my sadness for months, as winter deepened and darkened and eventually turned into spring. We emptied the trailer and sold it, planting a flower garden where the house had been. Late the following summer, I walked through the garden picking wildflowers; cosmos and zinnias and gladiolas burning against the stark, endless blue sky. That sky is something I miss whenever I feel homesick. How it stretches on for miles over cornfields, no towering buildings or smog to obscure it. How clean that sky felt. The wildness. The heartache.

***

"Can you believe it's been fifteen years since mom passed away?" my grandmother says. We are standing in my parents' kitchen on a warm September day. I'm home for the dual purpose of a work trip and to visit my family. Autumn is my favorite season, but I'm visiting a few weeks before the leaves turn crimson and sunsets burn like oil paintings. We are in the belly of a late summer heat wave and everything about being home had me feeling nostalgic: the tree frogs chirping in the swamp at dusk, the American flag hanging in the garage where I sit on the tailgate of my father's pickup truck as he stokes charcoal on the grill.

"No," I answered my grandmother, "I really can't." A lot has changed since the trailer was pulled away. The garden is full and flourishing. The giant elm tree that stood in the back yard is gone now, and with it, the tree swing. My father is not one to get lost in nostalgia, and he harrumphs, "It's a bad deal," and I assume he means that death is a bad deal, mostly, for the people like *us* who aren't dead yet. "None of us is getting out of here alive ya know."

"Oh, Todd don't say things like that," my grandmother admonishes. The closer you are to death, the harder it is to joke about.

My father waves his hands in the air and turns on his garage radio. He also has a garage TV, a garage heater for the winter, a garage fan for the summer, and a garage oven, where he makes fries with potatoes dug from the garden. "Ladies love Country Boys," blares through the radio speakers. "You know this song?" he asks me, as if he were a teacher quizzing me on a math problem.

"Sure, I do," I say with some indignance.

"Just making sure. You know what," he pauses, grill tongs in one hand, an old John Deere hat sitting lopsided on his head, "I think you're a California redneck."

I laugh, because I know what he's thinking. It's easy to assume that the entire state of California is as densely populated as Los Angeles, but California is a hugely diverse state, with wide swaths of unpopulated land and plenty of people just like my father. There are rednecks everywhere.

"No really!" He says, "That could be a song. *California Redneck*. I'll get to writing that for you."

My grandmother sits on a wooden bench, laughing and shaking her head. My grandfather is next to her nodding off, his glasses slipping down his nose. My brother is coming over later with his wife, their baby, and their dog. The corn is high and nearly ready for harvest, the garden plump with ripe tomatoes, carrots, and bulging hills of potatoes. The air is still and so quiet I can almost hear it.

"*California Redneck,*" my father says again, more to himself than to anyone else, "I like that."

CANCER'S BEST FRIEND IS CANCER

My mother's name is Denise, middle name Diane. My father calls her DD, when he's happy, or when he's upset. "Well DD," he'll say, exasperated, "you have to *open* it first," as my mother tries, unsuccessfully, to shake parmesan over the top of a casserole. My mother is a woman who loves putzing around the kitchen, taking the time to make a lemon meringue pie, for example, or lasagne, or homemade bread.

"I'm going to get fat if you keep feeding me like this," my father complains, not unkindly.

"You better not, or I'll put you on a diet!" my mother retorts, moving the butter dish to the far end of the table where my father can't reach it.

My father rolls his eyes and looks at me in false aggravation, "See what I have to put up with" he says, chuckling roundly.

"Hey, keep me out of this!" I say, "I'm a neutral third party."

We're eating steak my father grilled over charcoal. "Always cook it too long," he grumbles, his head in his plate. My mother dug a hill of baby red potatoes that my father calls, *better than candy*. I picked and cleaned spinach and lettuce for a salad, topping it with carrots and radishes and broccoli, all from the garden as well.

My parents have spent every summer growing food, harvesting it, freezing it, canning it, pickling it and filling our dinner table with hand-picked produce. I learned that it is uncomplicated and economical to grow your own food. For mere dollars, we could order all the seeds we'd need to plant a huge, sprawling garden. We ate organic food before it was posh, and I spent many long hours barefoot, squatting to pick strawberries or sitting outside the garage with a huge silver bowl in my lap snapping beans or extracting peas from hundreds of hard, ripe pods.

My family ate dinner every night at the table, no TV or phones to distract us. Once my brother and I got a bit older, this ritual became somewhat hectic as we juggled my sports with his sports with any other number of after school activities. But for the most part, we all ate together as much as possible, until my senior year of high school, when my mother was diagnosed with cancer.

My maternal grandmother died of breast cancer when my own mother was only 23. I was 18 when my mother received her diagnosis, and it felt like history may be cruelly repeating itself.

It was early spring, and I came home late from a date with my cute but dull boyfriend, but I don't remember anything that occurred before walking into the house. My parents and brother were waiting for me, and even before I walked in the door, I knew something was wrong. All the lights were on, despite the late hour. *Did I do something wrong?* I thought.

"Sit down, hun," my mother said, as I entered the dimly lit living room.

I said *why*, and *what's happening*, and she said, *I have cancer*, and I said *How?* and she said *tests* and *surgery* and *chemo* and my whole body went numb. *It's going to be okay*, she said. But I didn't believe her.

It's going to be okay, said my boyfriend.

It's going to be okay, said my teachers.

It's going to be okay, said my friends and my coaches and my relatives. But that's just what everyone says when they don't know what else to say.

My mother was, and still is, the backbone of our family. It was my mother who made sure we ate dinner together every night, my mother who made sure all the bills were paid, sorted through the laundry, carefully wrapped Christmas and birthday gifts. My mother was the one who signed permission slips, brought us to the dentist, fought with insurance companies over medical bills, and made sure my brother and I had small college funds. I was certain that nothing was going to be okay, ever again.

Mom was sent to have surgery at the Mayo Clinic in Rochester, MN. My father stayed there with her for many days, and my grandparents took my brother and I to visit her on weekends. In my fog of numbness, I was carrying on as if everything were normal, studying for my senior year finals, going to track practice after school, texting my boyfriend before bed each night. I felt eaten alive by worry and heartache, which was especially hard when I came home each night to an empty house.

Instead of coming home and sitting down to dinner with my family, I was left to fend for myself. I stopped eating at all during the day because starving myself felt like something I could control. All of my willpower dissolved at night, when I attempted to pull myself out of my numbness by eating a *lot*. An entire box of cheerios, a feast of eggs and toast, a bag of chicken nuggets accompanied by a bag of frozen peas. I ate until my stomach hurt and guilt pooled sourly behind my earlobes. Then, I'd lock myself in our pink tiled bathroom and turn on the shower, but I wouldn't get in it. I'd turn on the sink, too, before sinking to my knees at the porcelain toilet. I learned exactly where to push the back of my throat so that all that food was no longer inside of me. When I was done, I cried.

***

Twelve years later, my mother is healthy and in remission. I'm in a waiting room at the Providence Women's Health Center in Mission Viejo, CA. The health center is painted pink, with silk floral arrangements on every unused tabletop. When I checked in, a kind woman with steely grey hair instructed me to fill out a form. When I handed her back my paperwork, she directed, "Wait here," and quickly scanned the pages clipped to a black plastic clipboard.

"You're awfully young," she licked her finger, flipped the page, and peered up at me over her black rimmed glasses.

"I have a family history," I tell her, "of breast and ovarian cancer."

She nodded, this was something she heard every day. "Wait here for the nurse," she said, "She'll take you back to undress and we'll have you out of here in no time."

As I waited, I took in my surroundings. There was a meditation room off to one side, calming instrumental music gently streaming from the speakers, and neat pink gowns that opened in the front. I was only there for a routine mammogram. It was my first mammogram, because I was 30 now, with a rich family history of cancer.

Having a rich family history is usually a good thing. A rich family history of attending Harvard, say, of working in the family real estate business, or of healthy procreation. Some families have rich histories of wealth and prosperity. Some families have rich histories of oppression or alcoholism or cancer. All of us never asked to be here or deal with any of it.

People with BRCA1 and BRCA2 gene mutations live with a much higher risk of developing ovarian, breast, and colorectal cancers, and my family has fought all of them, although my mother does not carry the gene. My mother's extended family were not wealthy, and treatment was not very sophisticated. The chasm between my doctor's office and their medical experience feels so wide that I can barely see the other side. As I waited for the nurse, I couldn't help but look backward a few generations to consider how far this has all come. I have a good job with good health insurance that covers precautionary treatments like yearly mammograms and pap smears. I don't have to wait until I'm incredibly sick to access treatment, and today's large machines worth hundreds of thousands of dollars can trace any abnormality with incredible precision.

My mother and her sisters have all had various breast or ovarian cancers as well. My mother was 47 when cancer was detected in her fallopian tubes, one of the rarest forms of ovarian cancer. I didn't know this at the time, but her cancer has a very high recovery rate; over 90% when detected before spreading outside the ovaries or tubes. But we didn't know if it had spread at first, and there is no doctor or research paper on this planet that can remove the fear that lives inside a rich family history. It was impossible to watch my mother in her sickness and not think of her mother, too, who never made it out of the darkness.

When you love someone who has cancer, and when you are physically close to that particularly cruel kind of suffering, you can't help but wonder if maybe your own story might run in parallel. Every time I see a new doctor, I'm struck by the weight of it; writing name after name, cancer after cancer, starting with those furthest away in time and ending with the closest person to me, my mother.

The woman at the check-in counter told me this was all precautionary. She asked if I was nervous. "You'll be fine," she reassured me as she looked down at my long list of my family members, "this doesn't mean anything." For a minute, I thought she may be right. I'm healthy and fit. I take good care of my body and try to take good care of my brain. But in my heart, I knew she was wrong. Family history can't mean nothing. Family is inextricable. Family is everything.

When I left, I was given a packet of information about genetic testing and a validation for parking that still required me to pay one dollar. As I drove home, I thought about how much money the hospital makes from all the people who pay a dollar to park as they have their bodies poked and prodded and tested and treated. Millions a year, I figured. When I got home, I added "mammogram" as a recurring event in my calendar so next May, I won't forget.

THE BIG A (ANOREXIA)

If you're a fan of running as a sport, you've likely heard of Molly Seidel. In 2020, she surprised the running world by placing second in the Olympic trials in what was also her first marathon attempt. Later, she brought home a bronze medal from the Tokyo games. Molly is a year younger than me and grew up in Wisconsin, too. She attended a small private school near Milwaukee that, like my school, was categorized as Division 3, the smallest athletic division in the state at the time. Because our schools were very far apart, we never raced one another except during state cross country or track meets. By the time I graduated, I had raced Molly a handful of times, and she always blew the competition so far out of the water that we all understood we'd be racing for second. I have half a dozen silver medals from state meets thanks to Molly, who was gracious and truly humble.

Every time I raced, I wore a silver necklace with a rainbow pendant that had the words "Follow Your Dreams," etched in cursive in the clouds at the rainbows' base. The two dreams that sustained me at that time were first, to win a gold medal at state and second, to earn a college scholarship.

I never did win a gold medal, but I did succeed in earning a scholarship. My high school made a big deal out of signing day, every student piling into the gym to watch as I signed my letter of intent to run for Bradley University, a small, private Division 1 school in Peoria, Illinois. I chose Bradley primarily because they offered me a full ride, and because the campus was small enough to not overwhelm me. With barely 6,000 students, Bradley felt like the perfect size.

My high school coach held a microphone, "Who here has been a teammate of Sarah's?" he asked the crowd of students. Dozens of girls stood up, and I swallowed hard at the public display. I wasn't sure if anyone there cared about signing day, but it didn't matter. I cared, because I was about to go to college without having to worry about money. This was a blessing in more ways than one, because soon after signing day, my mother was diagnosed with cancer.

As the spring semester of my senior year crawled along, my mother's sickness deepened, like the darkness before dawn. After spending weeks at the Mayo Clinic, she came home with a twelve-inch scar on her stomach. The cancer had not reached her lymph nodes, and the doctors were confident that with chemo, she would be okay.

My mother was not well for a long time. She was exhausted and gaunt, and while I emptied my stomach into the toilet each night, she struggled to eat anything. By the time the state track meet rolled around, my mother was depleted but determined to attend. "I don't want to miss your last track meet, sweetie," she told me.

My body was not responding well to starvation, binging, and purging. I was not in peak physical fitness going into the state track meet, but who the hell cared? I'd see my mother sitting in the stands and feel overwhelmed with gratitude that she could be there at all. At the same time, I was still overwhelmed with fear. Mentally, I was worlds away from the track, even as I rounded it more than a dozen times between three different races.

I ended my senior year state meet with two silver medals and one bronze. After my last race, I made my way up the bleachers to find my parents, wanting nothing more than to give my mother a hug. I found them chatting to my new college coaches, two lanky men with grinning faces. I didn't feel like smiling. "Great job out there Sarah!" they said, slapping my back and looking me up and down. I hated how their eyes critiqued my body, which was slower and softer than it had been just a few months earlier. Maybe they saw fatigue, or the puffiness around my eyes, or the hopelessness that had lain just beneath the surface of my skin for weeks. "Thanks," I mumbled, and wrapped my mother in a hug.

***

The summer before I left for Bradley was also the summer my mother lost her hair. Both my parents accompanied me to Bradley for orientation, a 3-day affair with little pomp and circumstance. We sat in a lecture hall, mingled with other students and parents, and met some of the incoming athletes who would be my future teammates. I met my best friend at orientation, a girl named Taylor from Nebraska, with long blonde hair, bright blue eyes, and a wide, welcoming smile.

My mother wore a scarf on her head because by then, she'd had enough rounds of chemo for her hair to begin falling out. Her head became a maple tree in early autumn, when the leaves turn, and begin dotting the ground beneath it. While we sat in a large lecture hall listening to people talk about college, what to expect and how to prepare, I noticed her maple tree was shedding its leaves faster, as if a windstorm had suddenly swirled up out of the depths of the soft chairs we sat on. My mothers' hair was falling out in clumps, and I felt a lump grow in my throat the size of a grapefruit. I couldn't swallow it but couldn't let it out, either.

My mother looked *good* without hair. For many years, she wore her hair long, below her shoulders. It fell in soft auburn curls, shining in the sunlight as she bent to pick peppers or carrots. She pulled it up in a ponytail and stuck it out the back of baseball caps when she had work to do outside, pushing a lawn mower back and forth or raking leaves into a wheelbarrow. I always thought my mother was the most beautiful woman in the world, and I imagine many young girls feel that way about their moms. I was scared when she first started losing her hair, but she was every bit as beautiful without it.

Throughout high school, I let my hair grow long, dying it dark with drugstore hair dye, cutting bangs that looked ridiculous, and wearing it in a ponytail most of the time anyway, as I bopped between early morning runs and after school practices. I cut it shorter my senior year and cut it even shorter again when I started running at Bradley. It was easier to have less hair when most of my days were spent running, showering, and running again.

Then, in the spring semester of my freshman year at Bradley, I saw a flier advertising an organization called St. Baldricks that raises money for childhood cancer. Bradley was hosting an event where people could fundraise and then have their head shaved.

I signed up, raised a meager amount of money, and sat in a chair on the grassy quad after one of my morning classes. A volunteer buzzed my head in quick, even strokes and I smiled broadly at her, "Thank you!" I said, wondering how I would look.

For weeks, I received compliments on my head, "you look great!" women would tell me, "I could never pull that off." In my cloud of disordered eating and self-loathing, I learned that other people found me pretty. I began wearing big hoop earrings and learned to lather sunscreen on my scalp. I kept my hair short for the next five years, to the chagrin of my then-boyfriend. I loved not having to worry about it and liked how quickly I could get ready. I felt like a man in that I had fewer beauty products, no bobby pins or hair ties floating around my bathroom. There was only one bottle of shampoo in my shower caddy; none of the leave-in conditioners or dry shampoos or hairsprays I'd needed before.

I liked that I'd broken the mold of what I thought women had to be, and I felt spunky and cool with my pixie cut. Plus, when my eating disorder settled deeply in my bones, my short hair didn't make such a mess when it started thinning. It was less noticeable and easier to hide. At one point, my hair seemed to stop growing much at all, and I extended the weeks between hair appointments. My stylist told me to take biotin to help it grow better. I said, "Sure thing," but didn't buy any. I knew why my hair was thinning, and it had nothing to do with Biotin and everything to do with anorexia. The story I told myself then, was that I cut my hair for my mom, but my reasons were more nuanced and selfish. I cut my hair to more easily hide my eating disorder, in plain sight.

MOVING DAY

When it was time for me to pack my things and head to Bradley, my mother was still sick and weak from her chemo treatments. It fell on my father to make sure I arrived in one piece with everything I needed. Peoria was a good seven-hour drive from home, and I stared out the window at the never-ending fields of corn as my father pushed heavily on the gas pedal. I had a suitcase full of clothing and some small knickknacks from home; a cat shaped music box that was once my great-grandmother's, a stack of photos of my family and friends, and the Bible I'd been given when I was confirmed.

My dad and I didn't talk much during the drive, and I wondered how things at home would be without me. I felt guilty for moving away in the middle of my mother's sickness, and even more guilty for my excitement. I had worked so hard for so long for the opportunity to run in college, and I was selfishly ready to feel normal again.

Years after I moved away from home, I would discuss these feelings of guilt with my therapist. She told me about compartmentalizing, how we block out traumatic or stressful events and feelings as a defense mechanism. I didn't know it at the time, but I compartmentalized well, sorting each of my struggles into neat mental filing cabinets that were color coded and alphabetized. My therapist told me that it's common for kids to feel conflicted about moving away, especially when things aren't going well at home. "It's not just that I was away from my family," I told her, "It's also that I was away from *home*."

We think that home is where your loved ones are, and that's certainly true. But my family is inextricable from the acres of land we worked on and loved. I wasn't just homesick for my mom, I was homesick for the farm and the decades of memories that were woven into the floorboards.

As my father drove to Peoria, I was trying not to think of home and trying not to think of what lay ahead of me at college. We arrived at my dorm and hauled all my belongings up to the eighth floor, where I would share a small, musky room with one of my new teammates. As we looked around at the empty room, I realized I'd forgotten something.

"I'm supposed to get a futon," I told my dad. My roommate and I each had bunk beds, and we had agreed to put a futon beneath one, and a TV beneath the other.

"Okay, where to then?" he asked, and after some deliberation we landed on buying a futon from Wal-Mart, or "Hell-Mart" as we liked to call it. When I had to accompany my parents on outings to Wal-Mart, my father and I would lag behind my mother, who had a shopping list tucked in her purse and who deliberated over which brand of paper towels were the most economical, down to the cent. To pass the time, my father and I came up with a game; if we saw someone in a matching sweatsuit, we'd get one point. A stained shirt was also worth one point. A butt crack or general belligerence, double points.

After we found the futon, we walked around Wal-Mart for a while, my father buying me some screwdrivers and a hammer, "Just in case." He wanted to buy me food, but all I really wanted was a giant bag of carrots, "Is that all?" he asked doubtfully. I thought I hid my eating disorder well, but I didn't. As my entire family gently nudged me to eat, I doubled down on my restriction, citing my blossoming running career as the reason for my discipline.

"Sure thing dad," I answered, "I have everything I need." I imagine my father felt sad on the seven-hour drive back home. Maybe he cried just a little bit. After the lights went out that first night on campus, I cried too, because I missed my father, and I was scared for my mother, and my life was so strange and so new.

My high school coach was a man I looked up to, who knew when to push me and when to pull me back. He knew, for instance, that I would run myself into the ground and needed someone to slow me down. My new coaches at Bradley knew very little about me or about any of my new teammates. They came to Bradley with a stated mission of turning the program from a ragtag group of okay runners to a nationally competitive team, which was admittedly no small task. I was part of their first recruitment class, and I knew from the start that they would push me hard. I relished the idea of running faster and training harder than I ever had.

Training didn't start when we arrived on campus that fall though, it started in the summer. They sent us a training program complete with day-to-day running plans, weight-lifting exercises, and nutrition advice. The training was nothing I hadn't already seen, mostly base building runs and cross training. Harder efforts, like tempo runs and speed work, would come later. The nutritional advice they gave us was unsophisticated at best. *Avoid cheese*, it read. *Avoid eating after 8 p.m. Have fruit for dessert. Remove sodas and processed foods.* The advice was dull and probably pulled from the front page of Google or Runner's World Magazine. It was centered around what not to eat, instead of what we should have been eating. I was underwhelmed and a bit disappointed; I was expecting something more rigorous or maybe, more restrictive. I already wasn't eating cheese, dessert, or processed foods.

During the first weeks of practice, I came to understand something about my new coaches that had not been obvious when they were recruiting me. They were *obsessed* with leanness. They talked at length about maintaining our "fighting weights," instructed us not to eat "bad things," and told us to seek nutrition advice from our weightlifting coaches who also were not credentialed dietitians. I was already on board with being lean, so I didn't exactly mind this singular focus. During my Freshman year, however, I relaxed my stringent attitude toward food. My mother was in recovery, and being around my new teammates relaxed and emboldened me. I didn't feel the need to control my food, or my life, so heavily.

In part because I was more relaxed and happy, I had a successful Freshman season, exceeding my coaches' expectations, or so they told me. I'd finished the year making the All-Conference teams in cross-country, indoor track, and outdoor track. After my freshman season was over, I was physically exhausted, my ferratin (iron) levels dipping dangerously low. I hadn't binged or purged since the previous summer, and after our team doctor prescribed a liquid iron supplement, I started to feel strong and confident in my body. But, as my times grew faster, so did the pressure to perform. With that pressure came a host of expectations that I wasn't expecting. If I was going to be a fast long-distance runner, my coaches told me, I had to look the part.

***

The summer after Freshman year, I returned home to the farm to work full time at the bank where my mother worked as the Human Resources Manager. My job was to process loans and purge old files from the basement. Working full time, keeping up my training, and maintaining a social life took a toll on me. A combination of over training, sleep deprivation, and lazy eating got the best of me, and I gained about ten pounds over the summer. In trying to do everything, I burnt myself out before the season even started.

When I got back to campus that fall, my coaches were open in their disappointment. It was time for me to get back down to my "fighting weight," they said. Other women on the team were growing thinner, while I had committed the cardinal sin of gaining weight. I was shocked at how small my best friend had become. Her cheekbones jutted, her shorts sagged, and her ribs showed through her uniform.

In comparing myself to my friend, I felt a strange mixture of shame and pride. Shame, because she was doing something right that I was so obviously doing wrong, and pride because I had made good money that summer, enough to get me through the school year with just a part time tutoring job. I had let myself slip, but I had also set myself up to be able to focus on my training during the school year. My need for control had transferred from my body, to money, and in stark contrast to most students at Bradley, I meticulously counted my pennies.

"Doesn't she look fit?" my head coach said. "If you could just drop some weight, you might start running faster, too." I agreed with them because I felt like I had to, and recommitted myself to becoming small, again.

One day, the coaches called me into their offices for a meeting about my race weight. "Mac," one of them said, addressing me by my nickname, "what do you think your race weight is?" When I just stared at him blankly, he tried a different angle, "how much did you weigh last year, when you made the All-Conference teams?"

"Gosh, around 135 I think" I answered. My body has always been naturally muscular, a fact that I often hated. My legs were especially damning, my calves too big for skinny jeans and my thighs required a size larger than my waist. At 135 pounds and standing 5'4", I was a size four and often felt too large for my sport.

"Okay great," my coach answered. "What do you weigh now?"

"Just over 140," I answered. I knew because we were weighed every week in the weight room. My clothes still fit fine, but I could tell they did not like my answer.

My coach paused, "What do you think about this…what do you think about trying to get under 130? Not too much, but enough to make you faster."

I agreed because that was all I could do. They didn't tell me how to lose weight, so I looked around and did what I saw my teammates doing.

For dinner, we ate large salads. We routinely discussed food, grew hangry on long bus trips, and watched what each other ate, emulating each other's habits. My roommate and I took to making lunch in our dorm room because the cafeteria food was "unhealthy." I was consumed with getting smaller, so I reverted to old habits and started starving myself again. I would sit in the library, staring at my books, drinking coffee, and listening to the gurgling of my stomach. Restriction became a twisted game, and I'd force myself to wait until noon to eat a small dish of cheerios, slowly sucking on each small, round O.

After chatting with my coaches, I resolved to do anything to gain a competitive edge. There was a CVS across the street from campus and I started buying over the counter appetite suppressants, diuretics, and fiber pills. They worked at suppressing my hunger in the short-term, but I'd end up bloated, or battling a migraine, or fighting diarrhea.

Sometimes, my body would rail against me, hunger too strong to be undeniable, and I would binge uncontrollably, eating crackers and raisins and pop tarts in my dorm room until my stomach was close to bursting, only to empty everything into one of many toilets. I liked the bathroom on the first floor of Geisert Hall, because it was a single-use room and there was enough noise outside to drown the sound of my retching. I liked the basement of Williams Hall because the bathrooms were often empty. Sometimes, if another girl happened to be in a neighboring stall, I'd joke about being hungover and she'd lend me some Tums saying, "We've all been there."

***

My sophomore year cross-country season, I lost fifteen pounds and ended the season with faster times than ever before. I loved how my uniforms fit my new, smaller body, and I loved how my coaches praised me for how "fit" I looked. When I went home for Christmas break, I went back to work at the bank. I'd run before work and go to a gym across the street after. All I did was work and workout and starve myself. I wasn't happy and not even a little bit celebratory. On New Year's Eve, I worked and went to the nearly empty gym. I ran on a treadmill until the lights blinked twice, signaling that the gym was about to close. I arrived back on campus even lighter than when I'd left, feeling like I'd won a small victory by not gaining weight over the holidays.

I didn't understand what was happening at the time, but my eating disorder was spiraling. I became obsessive about food and about my body. I was often so tired that I couldn't concentrate on school, and running was becoming a lot harder and a whole lot less fun. My coaches reiterated countless times that I was doing the right thing "Runners look different," they said. "Runners are thin. It isn't unhealthy, it's just how runners need to be." They didn't know how I dropped the weight or kept it off, and they also didn't care. It wasn't their job to care, it was their job to make us run fast, and an unfortunate side effect of the collegiate running system is that many young women break their bodies before they ever reach their physical peak.

Because I was suddenly very light, I was temporarily very fast and then, I was injured. This is an unfortunately common cycle: a young woman will drop a lot of weight, maybe 20 pounds. She drops more weight than she should, and she's rewarded with huge PR's (personal records) and the fleeting attention of her coaches, competitors, or teammates. She is not stronger or healthier. In fact, she's weaker and less healthy, but nobody talks about that. Everyone praises her for how thin and "fit" she looks and for how fast she is running. Her uniform is baggier, her body invincible. For a while, she rides a euphoric high. Maybe she wins a few races, and maybe, for a season, she is the person to beat. Then, she always, inevitably, gets hurt. Maybe it's a stress fracture or a torn ligament or some unidentifiable illness. She's out for a season or two and even though she fights hard, she doesn't come back to compete at the same level she ran at pre-injury. Sometimes, she doesn't come back at all.

IOU

My brother is seventeen months older than me and infinitely wiser. As small children, we looked like we could have been twins though our dispositions couldn't have been more different. My brother was calm and curious, always taking things apart to figure out how to put them back together. I was loud, impatient, and energetic, easily upset and easily entertained, so long as I had space to run. Luckily, the farm we grew up on provided an endless outdoor playground, and my brother and I spent long hours outside, riding bicycles, playing in the mud, helping my parents rake leaves or dig potatoes from the garden.

My brother was the first one to lose a baby tooth, and my parents told us about a magical fairy that dances through the night to gather teeth from beneath the pillows of boys and girls, leaving money in exchange for a molar or two. I was in awe, wondering what this magic fairy looked like. Tinkerbell? Thumbelina? What does she want with the teeth? What does she *do* with them? Every time I lost a tooth I placed it carefully under my pillow, vowing to stay awake long enough to catch the fairy doing her dirty work. I could never fight my drowsiness, sleep tugging at my eyelids like a brick drifting to the bottom of a pool. I never caught the fairy red-handed, but she always came.

One morning though, after my brother slipped a tooth under his pillow, the tooth fairy *didn't* leave money. Instead, she left a note that read, "IOU," which my mother explained meant that the fairy was out of money and would leave some the following night. My brother and I weren't concerned about a missing dollar, but we were concerned with deciphering the tooth fairy's handwriting. *Maybe*, we whispered to each other, she was someone we *knew*.

We lived a lower-middle class life, and waiting for payday was just part of it. Later, when my brother and I were in high school, my parents both lost their jobs in the 2008/2009 economic recession. Life as we knew it was constricted and clouded with an unspoken scarcity. Thanks to my mother's astute budgeting we didn't lose the house, the outbuildings, or the farmland, rich and expansive and full of mystery. We had a beautiful, drooling mutt of a dog and enough to get by. Most of all, I had a safe, loving family. A father who played basketball in the driveway. A mother who baked homemade bread, punching it down, letting it rise, punching it again. I had everything I needed because I didn't need much, and I still don't. When you get used to getting by on less, even modest increments of wealth feel like a lot.

Despite the richness of our lives, growing up with economic insecurity made me terrified of being poor. Watching my mother keep close tabs on every cent that came in and went out planted a seed of stress that blossomed with an undercurrent of uncertainty because I learned that nothing in life is safe, and nothing in life is certain.

I am not currently living in scarcity, but the memory of it still lingers. So many of us are closer to the bottom than we realize. Being economically disadvantaged is an experience some people will never understand or can't. But for every person living comfortably in the upper middle class there are dozens living near the poverty line. Our culture goes to great lengths to make money seem like it is everything, and it can make life significantly better. One of the blessings of my childhood is that money *wasn't* everything. My childhood was rich with love and laughter and the great, wild outdoors. I had so much already. The tooth fairy didn't matter.

The tooth fairy would not have been happy, though, with how I treated my teeth after I left home. I stopped seeing a dentist and started chewing gum to quell my hunger pains, grinding my teeth together as if air were a suitable replacement for food. I started drinking a lot of coffee and subsequently whitening my teeth. I started throwing up more often, my stomach acid burning my esophagus and eroding my enamel. After four years of neglecting my dental care, I finally went to a dentist. The state of my teeth embarrassed me, and I grated them together at night which caused my jaws to ache and pulsate.

The hygienist wore all white, with her long brown hair in two separate braids. When she saw my teeth, she seemed unsurprised, telling me, "You sure have been hard on this enamel. I'm going to give you some special toothpaste to use. Do you drink a lot of caffeine? Or a lot of alcohol?" Caffeine yes, alcohol, not really. When I did drink, I was so anxious about the calories in the alcohol that I wouldn't eat all day, and then it didn't take much for me to feel buzzed. This is colloquially called "drunkorexia" and refers to someone who restricts food calories to make room for calories from alcohol. One study found that 46 percent of college-aged women engage in this behavior, not because we are scared to drink but because we fear becoming fat, and that is a fear that starts *young*.

I was barely 12 years old when I promised myself that I'd never be fat. Ours is a culture at once obsessed with and afraid of food. Ours is a culture that is hyper-focused on bodies: their shape, their size, their attractiveness, their desirability. But what good is a hot body if it isn't strong enough to do anything worthwhile? What good is being conventionally attractive if you can't concentrate on anything else?

My hygienist underscored the symmetry of my face, my teeth, and my body, telling me, "You are such a pretty girl, you have such a pretty face. It would be a real shame to let your teeth fall apart." She prodded my gums tenderly with her metal scaler, "You don't want that, do you?" I didn't, but not for the reasons she was implying. I didn't want my teeth to get too messed up because I didn't want to pay to fix them. The economic scarcity I felt as a teenager still hummed healthily through my veins and I knew enough to know that medical debt can come quickly and remain debilitating. I wanted a nice smile, sure, but that was not my primary concern at the time. My primary concern was not eating, and my teeth were not a strong enough incentive to convince me otherwise.

***

"You have been *impatient*," my father says, "since the day you were *born*." I'm chatting with my parents over the phone years later, on a Sunday evening in February. It just so happens that I was born on my parents' fifth wedding anniversary, February 6th, 1993. My parents briefly recount the day they got married, a ceremony with little fanfare held in a sleepy countryside church in the dead of an icy Wisconsin winter. After the ceremony, they *drove* to Florida. It's worth noting that they did not fly because my father is not a man who trusts airplanes or who enjoys close physical proximity to strangers. Besides, a plane ride is so pedestrian. A drive is an adventure. Their honeymoon 36 years ago was the first and last time they will ever make that particular drive, "Oh jeezus Florida," says my father, "I never have to go back there, I'll tell ya what."

My mother was in labor for about 90 minutes before I entered the world, dark haired and screaming. People always tell me that I look like my mother, but my temperament is a carbon copy of my father's: impatient, easily annoyed, yet often amiable and witty. My impatience allegedly started at birth and only worsened from there. "I remember," my mother announces, "the first time I took you to the dentist." I vaguely remember it too, the dentist was an old man, white hair matching his white robe. The dental office was dark, with wood-paneled walls and a dental chair that scared the bejeezus out of me.

"You kicked and screamed and *wailed*," my mother says, "and the doctor still gave you a toy from that jar of his." My mother doesn't mention it, but my brother sat in the monster chair like a seasoned stoic and let the dentist poke around his mouth *quietly*. I didn't understand his composure then, and I don't understand it now. "I actually went to the dentist the other day," I tell my parents.

"Any cavities?" my father says.

"No," I answer, "but they did want to give me fluoride and I don't know…it just seems like I shouldn't need that anymore."

My father scoffs, "You don't need *fluoride*, what are you, *nine*?" I picture his face, his mouth slightly open and his head cocked to one side, like he always does when he's irritated by something.

My mother, ever the pragmatist, says, "You don't need that, dear. They used to treat your teeth with fluoride when you two were little because we have well water here. It's not treated with anything like the water you have now."

Oh, I think, and sigh. It seems like everyone, at every turn was trying to sell me something or swindle me out of my hard-earned money. It's a cruel lesson to learn that medical providers are not inherently trustworthy, and that fighting an insurance claim could take many hours, if not weeks, of frustrating phone time.

"They're all crooks! The lot of them," I say, and my father answers, "Ya know what, I couldn't agree more," with such poise and finality that all three of us knew the case was closed. I picture my mother rolling her eyes, sitting at the kitchen table in her robe. She could see herself in the bay window, snow shimmering across the lawn in wide blue swaths, the ice under the birdfeeder pocketed by seeds and the pronged footprints of cardinals, blue jays and chickadees. Just like a painting.

DR. BRILLE DE RAMIREZ

My freshman year of college, I didn't declare a major. Most of my brain was focused on running, and I didn't have a plan for my future career. I hadn't given it any thought and I honestly couldn't see that far ahead, like a lot of 18-year-olds. I vaguely knew that I wanted to be a writer, but hesitated to declare an English major because I didn't know how writing could turn into full time income. My first two semesters, I focused on getting my general credits out of the way, and my first college class ever was an introduction to Native American Literature, taught by a bright, spunky woman named Dr. Susan Brille de Ramirez.

"How many of you are Freshman?" she asked on day one, a wide smile stretching across her tanned and welcoming face. A smattering of raised hands answered her question.

"Very good. How many of you are in your first ever college course?" A few hands remained up, including mine. I was in the front row, eager to be back in the familiar shape of a desk. I knew how to be a good student and latched onto that as my life buoy in this wild, new college landscape. Dr. Ramirez looked directly at me and said, "Welcome! You are going to learn so much."

I sat in the front row for the rest of the semester because I was so engaged with what we were learning. Dr. Ramirez's classes often went long, but I didn't care. We read books by Sherman Alexie, Kimberly Blaeser, Simon J. Ortiz, Gordon Henry, and Joy Harjo. We learned about Native rituals and beliefs, and about how elders can impart wisdom not found in any book. We learned how many tribes fought to hold onto their ancestry after being tormented, disrespected, and abused. My high school was about as good as a small, rural public school in a low-income district could be, but I was not exactly prepared for an intense college course load. I spent large chunks of time at a table in the basement of the student center, sipping bitter Starbucks coffee with my feet tucked underneath me. I didn't love studying, and focused my time in order of interest, starting with my English and writing classes, moving on to history and art, and ending with math and chemistry.

I never liked chemistry, and I didn't understand why I *needed* to understand complex math like calculus or trigonometry. It hasn't been necessary in my life at all, but other things that we didn't learn in school *have* been. How to build credit, for one. How to apply for a car loan or an apartment. How to read the contracts you sign before buying a car or renting an apartment. How to find a good mechanic in a new city. How to invest. How to start a retirement plan. How to resolve roommate issues. How to file taxes. How to change a tire, cook a healthy meal, or any number of adult minutiae. Instead, I found myself forced to study subjects like organic chemistry, oceanography, and algebra that had no useful impact on my life and no bearing on my health or wellbeing. I scraped by in those classes, and in my sophomore year, declared myself an English major. Nothing else made sense. Nothing else was even remotely interesting.

Many of my friends and teammates bonded over their heavy courseloads. Most were studying biology or pre-med. Sometimes they poked fun at my major because it was considered useless and easy. But I wasn't learning things that had pretty, solid, black, and white answers. I was contemplating larger questions that have real implications but no *good* answer, like how language impacts how we see the world and how our perspectives and experiences influence our language. In one class, we made lists of slurs for women, then lists of slurs for men and debated the disparities. We argued over how much language mattered, and why. We read books about critical theories and learned to extrapolate our own ideas from those theories. We formed cohesive written arguments and sat in circles editing each other's writing and discussing how to make our own writing better.

We read books that were written a long time ago, and thus learned untaught history. We read Shakespeare because we had to. We learned how to write a good argumentative essay, how to write compelling business proposals and complete thoughtful narratives. We learned to communicate as clearly as possible within the limited confines of language, and that is a less tangible skill than engineering or calculus, but it's just as valuable. I loved my major, and I loved school when I was able to study what I wanted to study. I viewed education not only as a path to a good career but also as a path to becoming a more evolved, thoughtful, and humane person, and Dr. Ramirez heavily influenced how I conceptualized education.

Dr. Ramirez also quickly became one of my mentors. I took as many of her classes as I could, and she helped me work around my hectic athletic schedule to complete more than one independent study. When I ran into her at 3030, a local coffee shop, she would smile broadly and offer me a seat. We would talk for hours, both of us neglecting our work. Sometimes, she would help me through a tough problem, whether it was in her class or not. When I decided to stay at Bradley for a 5th year to fulfill my athletic eligibility and complete my Master's in English, she helped me write a plan of attack, which courses to take and when. She became the first woman ever to direct the English Master's program at Bradley, and instituted new, forward-looking courses that were met with resistance from some of her peers but were largely embraced by her students. In one class, she had us write ebooks and put them up for sale on Amazon, recognizing that digitizing the humanities was the only way to keep them alive.

Dr. Ramirez and I stayed in touch after I left Bradley, and the last time I saw her was the summer after I graduated, when I was back in town for a visit. I stopped by 3030 and she was there, the same as always, working away tirelessly on her laptop with a half-empty cup of coffee next to her keyboard. She asked what I was doing, how I liked Chicago, where I might want to end up or what I most wanted to do. She saw potential in me that I couldn't, at that time, see in myself. And I saw in her a version of a woman who was strong and sure of herself—who went after what she wanted without apology or complaint. So many of my teachers were men, and they were mostly good, but Dr. Ramirez was different because I saw elemental pieces of myself in her; the disagreeableness that so many of her peers disliked, but that made her respected and successful, the deep appreciation for art, her desire to give voice to people who were often left voiceless. And of course, the mere fact of her womanhood. Dr. Brille de Ramirez gave me confidence, but she also inspired me. I deeply wish I could tell her that now.

After I moved to California, we emailed a bit, and I didn't hear back from her for a while. One afternoon, as I sat in my office at the Orange County branch of the American Red Cross typing out a grant proposal, I saw a missing person's alert pop up on Bradley's Twitter page. Dr. Ramirez and her husband, who also worked at Bradley, were both missing. My hands stopped typing. My heart rate doubled. Dr. Ramirez was never late to class, ever. Fear is a living thing, and it crept up from the depths of my office chair that day, circling my windpipe.

The general sentiment online was not good. The news stories crumpled into one another, cruelty and heartache mashed together like gauze to a gaping wound. Dr. Ramirez and her husband were sleeping in their country home when their grown son, who they had adopted late in life, entered their bedroom and stabbed them to death. His reasoning was that he was "sick of his parents," but there really was no reason at all. Some called him evil. Some called him mentally ill. One of his friends helped. They dumped the bodies in a nearby river and freely admitted to the crime days later. Dr. Ramiriz and her husband fought back hard, according to police reports. There were signs of blunt force alongside stab wounds. I wondered what I'd last said to her. I wondered if she knew how much she meant to me.

Months after she passed, I wrote this poem and sent it to the Bradley Alumni magazine. I wanted her to know that she was loved.

You Are Going to Learn So Much
after Dr. Brill de Ramirez

If I had a dollar for each time you stopped me at a coffee shop
to chat for a minute that turned into an hour
I'd have enough cash to buy a beach front home
with huge bay windows facing the sunrise,
the same direction your office perched on the third floor
of the only building on campus that felt like home

you were the first person I ever heard say,
stories changed my life. stories saved my life
you were my first professor, literature
came to life in your eyes,
pulled me into a non-linear understanding of time

you taught me to pay attention to empty space
wrote at the bottom of my thesis *poetry is the art of silence.*
you always said yes to independent studies
office hours extra time to complete assignments
when my chest was constricted and anxious
you never said no to giving more

most people take, stacking boxes of belongings
around them like shields
you gave away swords
turned anger and hurt into learning and love

in the long spring days of Ramadan
you ate burritos at the front of an English class
all of us weary but wanting to learn
to read and speak and be heard
you were always so eager to listen

when I heard you'd gone missing
my heart sank like lead
when I heard you were dead
I closed the door to my office

sank to my knees and sobbed
my limbs turning numb
ears ringing the sound of your quiet hum

I miss how your laughter
skipped down the steps of Bradley Hall
where magnolia tress blossomed late into April
I want you to know
your echo is louder than the anger that stole you
your spirit is strong and tenacious
lovely and free and relentlessly kind

one day I will drive to the desert
write a poem in the sand and sign your name
pray to God you are safe now
promise to carry you with me
your spirit of iron
conviction like fire in my veins
you are so far away but I wanted to say,
thank you

HELP, I BROKE MY HIP

During my junior year of college, only a year after I dropped a good 20 pounds to become lighter and faster, I started feeling a lingering pain in my right leg. My entire leg felt hard to lift, and my power was suddenly gone. Sometimes my entire leg went numb, and nobody could determine the cause of my pain. For more than a year, I had managed to starve myself thin while avoiding injury. I was worried that my luck had run out and that I would be one of the injured girls leaning on crutches watching her teammates run free.

I went to the team doctor, who told me to rest. I saw a chiropractor, massage therapist, and a physical therapist. I had acupuncture done and spent an entire summer injured, unable to train. I grew increasingly depressed, not just because I was injured but because I didn't know how to fix it. My team doctor, who was herself frustrated at not being able to identify the cause of my pain, told me that maybe I was just "feeling things," and that sometimes, "we need to run through pain." Her words ignited a fury I didn't know I was capable of. My competitive nature held no space for weakness, and I knew my body. My pain was not fleeting. It moved in, built a home, and had no intention of leaving.

Nearly six months after the onset of my symptoms, I saw a different physical therapist, a man who was also a professor at Bradley. He immediately ordered an MRI with contrast, which would more easily show any small tears or injuries. His conjecture was a torn labrum in my right hip, and he was right. The team doctor texted me the results, and I fumed at her cowardice. The right and decent thing would have been to call me, like she had when she told me I needed to run through my pain. From then on, I avoided her with such astute intention that I don't recall ever having a conversation with her again.

I was flown to Vail, Colorado to the Steadman clinic for surgery from one of the best doctors in the business. I stayed there for seven days post-op for physical therapy, my parents hovering closely the entire time. After the surgery, I lay in bed for hours, unable to move my legs because they had given me too much anesthesia. After I regained the ability to move, the next order of business was re-learning how to activate my glutes and my hamstrings. My muscles had gone dormant, and I felt like a child who just discovered walking. Only a year before my surgery, I had been running as fast as I ever would. I struggled to grapple with my new, broken body, and doubled down on the one thing I felt like I could control: food.

Before I left for my surgery, one of my coaches warned me against eating too much. "It's easy to gain weight while you're injured," he said, "be careful not to let that happen." By now, I was accustomed to advice like this, and found it unsurprising, albeit normal, that his only concern would be my weight. I took his recommendation in stride and embraced my old habits: restriction, diet pills, purging. I don't remember many details of that trip because I was in a mental fog, exhausted and trying my best not to eat.

One night in Vail, a few days after my surgery, my parents took me out to a beautiful Italian restaurant for dinner. As soon as we sat down and looked at the menu, I started to cry. There was nothing on the menu that I could let myself eat; it was all rich and decadent and I was irrefutably overwhelmed by my entire situation; being in Vail, feeling isolated and lonely, feeling eons away from where I had been just one short year earlier, the pain in my body, and the overwhelming, constant, pain in my brain. My carefully constructed world was tipping on its axis, and I was entirely unable to right myself again.

When my parents dropped me off at the Denver airport, I was left to navigate the airport on crutches, and then in a wheelchair. I waited at the gate for more than two hours, my butt growing numb as I sat. I was the first to board the plane, and felt my hip tighten as I stood from the wheelchair and squirmed my way into a seat. The dull ache in my hip would persist for many months, and my physical pain became a convenient proxy for my mental anguish. The more my body hurt, the quieter my mind became. I didn't understand that this was anything but normal and anything but healthy.

When I returned to campus, I spent six weeks hopping to class on crutches and sleeping in a CPM (continuous passive motion) machine that extended my leg back and forth as I struggled to sleep. Months after my surgery, I was cleared to run again for one minute, my chest straining as my body struggled to adapt to being in motion. I had a long way to go if I wanted to reach my previous level of fitness. The difficult truth was that I never would. I never regained the speed I had, briefly, when I was starving myself thin, before my body broke.

One of the coaches from a rival school, who unsuccessfully recruited me back when I was a starry-eyed high schooler, spoke to me at an indoor track meet after I'd made my slow comeback. We were standing in the large oval of an indoor track, watching runners whiz by in a 1500 meter race.

"It's hard coming back," he said, his neck stretching toward me, "and Sarah, it's such a shame. You had so much potential."

I wasn't sure how to interpret his words. I wasn't offended because he was right. It *was* a shame. I *did* have so much potential. I just wasn't sure who had taken it away from me, or how to get it back.

When I was in second grade, my teacher cut a red heart out of construction paper and crumpled it into a ball before smoothing it back out. "When we hurt someone's feelings," she said, "their hearts grow a wrinkle. It might fade with time, but it's always there." My body, after I graduated, was full of wrinkles. Injuries and scar tissue; a fucked up digestive system and clinical malnourishment. Continuing to run felt impossible, so I took a break, entered therapy, and began the long, slow process of fixing my body and re-orienting my brain.

***

"I bought you some que-no-wa," my mother says, grabbing a bag out of the pantry, which was once an entryway closet. When I was in seventh grade, my parents decided that one bathroom was not enough for two teenagers and two adults. They hired a contractor who dug out an addition to the basement and worked his way up. The result was a spacious new entryway, second bathroom, and upstairs laundry room so my mother didn't have to trek up and down the stairs as she did load after load of laundry. The addition made the house feel new and twice as big.

"It's *quinoa*, mum," I gently corrected her. I'm visiting home during spring break of my fifth year at Bradley, and my mother is trying to make sure that I'm fed. I'm vegan, so I don't eat meat or cheese, which means I can't eat most of her signature dishes. Instead, I eat a big scoop of quinoa and vegetables, lying as I tell my family that I'm getting enough to eat, really, and it's actually quite good.

The conversation loops and roams, from work to school to the track season that still lay ahead of me. I wasn't quite done yet, but I was close, and I was tired. Fighting my way back from injury was slow and frustrating work, as I was sidelined time after time by small nagging pains. "You're still a big part of that team," my father reminds me as we sit around the dinner table. And he's right. I was no longer the fastest girl on the team, but I was still earning points at track meets and made the conference roster in cross country.

"I know," I say, "it just isn't the same." I meant that running wasn't the same, but it was so much bigger than that. Running didn't feel like flying anymore, it felt like a struggle. Every step came with pain somewhere in my body, sometimes a dull aching pain in my hip and sometimes sharp pain, traveling from my hip to my knees all the way to my ankles. My joy was gone, and my mother, sitting across from me, sensed my stark lack of enthusiasm. She put her silverware down and looked over at me.

"We're proud of you, honey," she says, and the conversation turns back to everyday matters; the dairy farm next door was expanding, a neighbor up the road is fighting cancer, the new pastor at church gave a hell of a sermon, insurance is still sending medical bills for my surgery. No one knows the depth of my physical discomfort or mental distress, and I was damned if I'd ever admit it.

WORK SUCKS

The summer between my Sophomore and Junior years of college, I applied for an internship at an auto insurance company. My sophomore year was a good one, in all the arbitrary ways I measured and thought about life. I dropped 20 pounds and was riding my momentary high, running faster than ever. My clothing hung loosely on my skinnier frame, and I felt validated in my belief that starving myself worked. I had a new boyfriend named Chad who was charming and funny and sweet (most of the time). I was earning straight A's in all my classes and finally declared my major. When things go well, it's easy to expect them to keep on going well forever, a delusion that's as easy to slip into as shrugging on a coat. Things never stay good or bad forever because things never, ever, stay the same.

After deciding to stay in the sprawling metropolis of Peoria over the summer instead of returning home to the farm, I drove myself to the insurance office for an interview, dressed in my one pair of black slacks and a button-up shirt from Ross. Did I think I'd ever become a car insurance agent? Never. But the job paid well and was predictable. It's easy to crave predictability too, especially when living in the chaos of an eating disorder. It wouldn't take me long to learn that predictability meant something much worse–boredom.

Anyway, I applied for the job, interviewed, and then received a rejection letter in the mail the following week. I wasn't in college that long ago. Email existed, as did phones. For some reason, the letter felt especially stinging. The idea of someone writing my address, adding a stamp, and licking the envelope closed felt both personal and astoundingly avoidant.

The man who interviewed me wore a light gray suit that made his pale skin and thinning blond hair look even more pale and even more thin. He told me he moved to Peoria from Florida, a state which he hated with undue passion, "too many old people," he said, "can't go out to dinner anywhere without encountering a sea of gray heads." I suppressed a small grin, thinking of a sea of elderly folks swarming a China buffet. Then, this man with thinning blond hair and crooked front teeth looked me dead in the eye and said, "What do you want to do with your life? What do you *plan* on *doing* with your…" he glanced down at my resume, "English degree."

I was twenty years old and had no idea what I wanted to do with my life, so that's exactly what I said, "I don't know," I answered, too truthfully. "Did you think you wanted to run an auto insurance office?"

"District," he corrected me, underscoring the fact that I didn't know about the other two branches he supposedly managed.

There was not an ounce of my being that wanted the job, but receiving the rejection letter in the mail of all places left me feeling immensely sad and more than a little bit angry. As I always did whenever I needed to complain, I picked up my cell phone and called home. My father answered. "Hey honey," he said, "How ya doin?" My father is a man who likes working with his hands, and he's always, no matter the weather, outside. He was outside that day when I called, tending to the tender young plants in his vegetable garden.

I was crying and could not hide it. I was about to have big feelings. "I didn't get the job," I choked out, in between sobs.
"Ohhh honey. That's alright, isn't it? You're going to find something."

"But I really thought the interview went *well*," I protested, knowing full well that the interview had *not* gone well. And then, the worst revelation, "I don't understand why they didn't choose me."

After a beat, my father simply said, "You might not ever know. But I'm sure you'll find something. Life has a funny way of working out, ya know."

I both loved and hated that my father was right. "Thanks Dad," I sniffled, and then I walked outside, revved up my tan Buick Lesabre, and drove around town looking for "Help Wanted" signs. I filled out applications at a diner, a Smoothie King, and a grocery store. Smoothie King offered me a part-time job, and the diner hired me for Saturdays only, 5 a.m. to 2 p.m. At Smoothie King, I could make myself one smoothie for every 4-hour shift. At the diner, I could drink all the coffee I wanted and none of the cash tips would be reported as taxable income. My rent was only three hundred dollars a month, and I usually earned my rent in one weekend.

Weeks after the auto insurance rejection letter hit my mailbox, I received a call from their office. "Sarah," the district manager said a little too brightly, "how are you?"

"Fine," I replied skeptically, wondering what this man wanted from me.

"Good," he said curtly, before cutting to the chase, "the person we offered the job to backed out and frankly, I think we made a mistake. Would you reconsider coming on board for the summer?"

By then, I had already started at Smoothie King, where I ran around manically, churning out smoothies, restocking inventory, and cleaning blenders. I made a dollar less an hour than the insurance company offered, but I had pride. I also kept a running mental tab of all my income and expenses, and that extra dollar tempted me, just for a moment, before I smiled into my phone, "No thank you," I said politely, "I've already acquired employment."

The following summer, the insurance company once again offered me a job, and this time, I took it. Instead of blending smoothies and chopping fruit, I was punching numbers into a computer system and twiddling my fingers behind a desk. Instead of moving around all day, I was stuck sitting for eight hours straight. Instead of interacting with customers I was interacting with a screen, and

I hated it. I had to wear business clothes and deal with people filing insurance claims. I had to be there by 8am and take a mandatory hour-long lunch break. It was a lonely and depressing place, and I missed the busyness of the smoothie shop.

I wanted the insurance job *so* badly, but it remains one of the most tedious and terrible jobs I've ever had. I wasn't pursuing what I needed, but rather, what I thought I wanted. I didn't know that I had goals, or what they would be, but I knew office work wasn't it. That was a lonely summer filled with boredom and listlessness. A summer of isolation and quietude. A summer that offered so much, but somehow, I took so little. The best part of that summer—the best part of *any* of my college summers—was a writing conference in a tiny town in Ohio called Yellow Springs.

***

"Your verbiage is clever, but sometimes verbose," my instructor wrote at the bottom of the packet of poetry I'd sent him prior to the start of the workshop. His name was Herbert Woodward Martin, a kind man with soft, yellowing eyes. Professor Martin was in his eighties with a strong and sturdy voice, like a worn-in but well-crafted canoe. He wore tailored suits and enunciated clearly.

"Here," he said, pointing to one of my poems entitled, "Breakfast of Champions."

"See this line? You add words to make it sing-songy, which probably helps you remember the poem, and which might make it good for oral performance." He paused for a moment, "but a written poem is different. Consider my edits and we'll talk about them tomorrow."

That poem begins,

My breakfast of champions
is a sugar cube dissolved in earl gray tea
and a teaspoon of cream

I slide into skinny size 0 jeans
with room to take up less
my stomach is a beast with razor teeth
I calm him with cups of tea
he pounds at my ribs counts all 24 of them
tight beneath skin I'm never comfortable in

I wrote this poem, and several others, as I was admitting to myself that I had an eating disorder. These were scary poems to write, because I was ashamed of my brain and very uncomfortable in my body. One thing that is typically misunderstood about eating disorders is that they're usually not all about food or bodies. My eating disorder gave me a weird semblance of control and a convenient outlet for my perfectionism. One night at the conference, I had a nightmare where I heard what seemed like dozens of voices screaming. The screams felt like they were all around me and there was nowhere to escape or hide. Even when I woke up, I still felt like I could hear them, my ears ringing, from *what*, I wasn't sure. That's how pervasive an eating disorder is: a constant noise that's sometimes a dull ring and often, a horrifying scream.

When I arrived in Yellow Springs, I checked in at a quaint bread and breakfast. The man at the front desk was the owner as well as the chef as well as a bike mechanic, "There are bikes out front you can use," he said. "I cleaned them up myself this morning. I'll give you a helmet and lock if you need em."

He wore a long-sleeved flannel shirt, despite the sticky Midwest air. I accepted this offer and hopped on a bright red bike, complete with a dainty wicker basket. I rode into town, surprised by the pedestrians walking around barefoot, the man outside a coffee shop playing a ukulele, the vegan food stores and recycled clothing shops. I'd inadvertently fallen into a hippie enclave in the middle of Ohio. Everyone was friendly, and I found myself tasting what life could be like if I weren't chained to my eating disorder. I could make friends with strangers. I could eat fro-yo at noon. I could explore a new city on a bright red bike, powered by my own two legs.

Yellow Springs has become infamous because Dave Chapelle lives there. When I visited Yellow Springs in the summer of 2015, I didn't know who Dave Chapelle was. I'd applied to this writing workshop on a whim and was surprised when I won a scholarship to attend. Dr. Kevin Stein, my poetry professor and Illinois poet laureate, helped me access funds from a small pool reserved for conferences in the English Department. My room at the bread and breakfast would be covered by these funds, and the scholarship covered the workshop's tuition. All I had to do was *get* there.

I drove the five hours from Peoria to Yellow Springs straight through, only stopping once for gas. The first morning of the conference, I woke up early to do a workout in my room, following along as a YouTuber took me through a series of split squats and jumping squats and pushups and jumping jacks. Halfway through my workout, the telephone rang. Not my cell phone, but the phone that was in the room on a wooden nightstand next to the bed. The phone you're only supposed to use for room service or to request a wakeup call. I ignored the ringing, throwing myself into my jumps and squats with even greater determination. The phone rang again. Again, I ignored it. The phone rang a third time, and I finally grabbed it, rolling my eyes.

"Hey," came the voice of the bread and breakfast owner/chef/bike mechanic, "are you jumping around or something? I'm getting complaints from the room beneath yours." My face flushed, even though he couldn't see me.

"Yes," I replied, looking out the window at a crisp, cloudless sky. "Yes, I am. I'll uh, quiet down."

The man on the other end of the line burst out laughing. "Alright then, have a wonderful morning," he said, and I heard the phone click back into the receiver.

After that, I decided to take my morning workouts outside. For the entire week, I would run some mornings with no thought as to how far or fast I went. Due to my bum hip, I ran a bit lopsidedly and it always hurt, but I didn't care. I relished the freedom of being in a new place and exploring the single lane country roads and dewy grass fields, my shoes growing heavy with water, the fresh air kissing my lungs like a heartache.

My days were full at the conference, with guest speakers and breakout sessions and editing sessions and endless conversations with other writers. I smiled more often that week than I had the entire summer.

On the last day of the conference, my peers chose me to do a reading. I stood at a podium in front of a large crowd and didn't feel any of the fear or anxiety I normally did in front of people. I'd rehearsed my poems so many times that I knew them by heart, and as I performed, I felt both naked and brave. I wrapped up my pain in neat little poems that left the audience silent at first, before they erupted in applause. My face flushed as I went back to my seat. A woman seated nearby grabbed my hands to say, "You did *beautifully.*"

When I arrived back in my normal life at the insurance company, I was suffocatingly depressed. I wanted to be back in the woods of Ohio where fireflies lit up the ditches at dusk and where writers gathered to make sense of the mysteries of language and life. I slowly lost the magic of that summer, bit by golden bit until all that was left were memories and a faded packet of poems with handwritten notes from Dr. Martin, "*Sarah,*" he wrote, "*you have come so far in such a short span of time. Your poetry is important. Please, keep writing.*"

***

I wrote "Breakfast of Champions" post hip surgery, before my return to running. My recovery plan consisted of extensive physical therapy and stationary biking with little to no resistance. Eventually, I could integrate non-weight bearing exercises into my routine, like aqua jogging or the elliptical machine. I would go to Bradley's student rec center with my swimsuit and a blue floatation device that sat around my waste. There, I would float in the deep end of a heavily chlorinated pool, pedaling my legs in a running motion for an hour or more at a time. It was mind numbingly boring. Sometimes, the lifeguards would play music. Sometimes, I would stare at a white brick wall in silence and think.

Eventually, I was able to upgrade out of the floaty and simply jog in place in the water. Because I was severely under-nourished, I could easily spend the entire hour thinking about food. One evening, my friend Taylor asked me to go to a local fro-yo shop. "After your swim session," she said, "I just need something sweet, and we haven't gone in forever." She was right, we hadn't gone in forever. I avoided social occasions centered around food, and I felt compelled to say yes. She cared about me, and I cared about her, but my surgery and eating disorder left me feeling isolated from everything any normal college aged student cared about. "I'll be there by 7," I told her and hobbled off on my crutches to go aqua jog.

The sky outside was already dark, and streetlights shined through the high pool room windows. I aimlessly kicked my legs and pumped my arms and thought about food. So much of my spare time was spent thinking about food, building Pinterest boards of recipes I never intended to cook just so I could look at photos of rich, decadent meals and sweets. As I stared at the white brick wall, I thought of all the food I used to love, but never allowed myself to eat anymore: my mother's casseroles, sweet, crunchy breakfast cereals, juicy, plump strawberries, sweet corn, peanut butter sandwiches, pasta, burgers. I fantasized about what kind of fro-yo I would have later. I hadn't eaten all day, and I promised myself I'd only fill the big paper cup a quarter of the way. Maybe I'd get caramel and chocolate. Or maybe I'd stick with plain vanilla and add sprinkles, like I always did when I was little and the Schwann's man would park his large truck in our driveway and deliver frozen fish and ice cream. I loved the tiny cups of vanilla with colorful sprinkles on top. I'd let the cups melt a bit and mix the sprinkles in until all the colors mixed into an odd, murky gray. Kick, kick, pump. Kick, kick, pump.

My great-grandmother kept those ice cream cups on hand during the long summer months when my brother and I raided her freezer for snacks. Food is just one of many ways people say, "I love you," and I thought about how actions can be more potent than words. Sometimes, actions *are* words. My mind wandered back to breakfast cereal, how my mother always bought the healthy stuff: Wheaties, Cheerios, Raisin Bran, Shredded Wheat, and sometimes, if they were on sale, Honey Bunches of Oats or Multi Grain Cheerios or Kix. Now, there were so many options in the cereal aisle that I gave up buying any—the vast quantities and confusing nutrition labels were enough to frighten me away. Kick, kick, pump. Kick, kick, pump.

The water was warm, and tiny beads of sweat broke out on my forehead.

"My breakfast of champions isn't anything," I thought. I had a habit of drinking cup after cup of coffee or tea to fill up my stomach and ease my hunger pains. The caffeine helped me feel alert and momentarily full, but it also made me shaky, frazzled, and cold. *"My breakfast of champions,"* I thought, *"is coffee with no cream. Or a sugar cube dissolved in earl gray tea and a teaspoon of cream."*

I kicked a little harder as I continued to form a poem in my brain, my creative energy giving me a minor adrenaline boost. My creative high lingered until I arrived at the yogurt shop, Taylor waiting patiently out front. She smiled broadly, "I'm so glad we're doing this!"

I ate a tiny cup of yogurt that night, plain vanilla with colorful sprinkles and bits of crushed up waffle cone. Later, I lay in bed and wondered if the yogurt would show itself on the scale the next morning. I wrote down the first few lines of my poem, which I would flesh out in the coming days. Eventually, I would take that poem to my poetry workshop and read it in a circle of my classmates, who were kind enough to understand that the darkness in that poem was a darkness deep within me.

They gave me feedback and edits, and my friend Hannah, who sat to my right, squeezed my hand, and whispered, "I love this poem, and I love *you*." With that poem, I cracked a wedge into my eating disorder that would one day crumble and disintegrate completely.

ROCK BOTTOM

My first therapist worked in Bradley's on campus mental health center. I was living with my boyfriend Chad by then, sharing a cheap but quirky apartment right off Main Street. Living off-campus was liberating because unlike most living units on campus, I could close a door and be in a room all by myself. I could boil water on my own stovetop and do laundry in a rickety washing machine that was not communal. Life in our apartment also made hiding my eating disorder simple and straightforward. I could order diet pills, laxatives, and appetite suppressants on Amazon with just a few clicks and one swipe of my finger. Most days, Chad worked late at a local running store, so I received the packages before he came home with plenty of time to hide them. I was so used to hiding that I grew lackadaisical or maybe I wanted to get caught. Either way, one late winter evening, Chad caught me ordering diet pills on my phone. His normally perky face went dark, "Sarah, what are you *doing*?" he asked. I looked down, unsure what to say.

"Nothing," I lied, but it was obvious that he didn't believe me.

He took my hand and gently squeezed, "I think you might have a problem. Those aren't good for you," he said, gently pointing at my phone screen.

Chad and I had a contentious relationship, punctuated by jealousy and poor communication and eventually, resentment. Despite his anger and my acquiescence, he could be disarmingly sweet and charming. It's hard to leave someone who is bad for you when most of the time, they don't *feel* bad, and something about how gentle Chad was that night broke a dam inside of me. It was easy to be hard when *he* was being hard. It was easy to not care about myself when he didn't, either. But the care and the gentle concern in his eyes unnerved me and I finally let myself cry, the self-hatred and fear I'd held inside of me for years free to break loose.

As my face contorted in an ugly cry, Chad looked at me hard, turning my face into his. "You need help," he said. "Do it for *us*."

I knew he was right, that I did need help. But I also knew I couldn't get help for *us*, I'd have to do it for *me*, and I'd have to do it because *I* wanted to get better. As quickly as I'd melted into his embrace, I felt myself grow icy again, and sat up straight, leaning away to put real and metaphorical space between us.

"Call the health center," Chad said, "or request an appointment online, you don't even have to call." He looked me in the eyes, "please?"

And much to my own surprise, I did.

A few days later he walked me to the health center, swarms of students milling about the campus, my brain so consumed with anxiety that I didn't notice or try to avoid the students walking past me. A girl in black combat boots whacked my shoulder with her book bag and I didn't even flinch. Chad walked me to the door before posting up in a nearby café, drinking coffee and working on his laptop while I admitted my deepest, darkest secrets to a kind woman in a floral print skirt.

I told her everything: how I'd started binging and purging years ago, right after my mom was diagnosed with cancer. How I nurtured a seed of hatred for my body and let it grow, and now, didn't know how to stop it. Its roots felt too deep, too strong. I told her how I felt separate from my body, as if it were not my own. How my coaches condoned any behavior that made me shrink, how they weighed us in front of everyone and measured our body fat percentages. How they controlled what we ate on team trips and consistently shamed our bodies. How my body broke because I abused it for too long. How it didn't make me feel good to starve but it did make me feel like I had some sort of purpose.

I told her how I didn't know what I wanted to do with my life, just that I wanted it to matter. How I hadn't even thought that far ahead because all I could think about was not eating and running and throwing up and the constant, sharp pangs of hunger that prevented me from sleeping each night. I told her how ashamed I felt, how I couldn't tell anyone that I had this problem, and that she was the first person I'd ever told. I cried and blew my nose into dozens of tissues, my hands clenching and unclenching, my pain rolling out of me in soft, undulating waves. I don't know how long I talked, but I felt relieved once I was done.

She looked at me with an unreadable expression and said a few things. First, she said, "You have been very brave today," which made me roll my eyes. I didn't feel brave, I felt gutted, like an overripe avocado being scooped into a bowl and mashed into guacamole. But then she said, "Your coaches have not had your best interests at heart. Unfortunately, you're not the first college athlete this has happened to." And finally, she said, "If you want to get better, you *can*. *Do* you want to get better?"

I nodded, looking at her miserably, even though her verbiage made me defensive. You don't agree to getting better unless you can agree that something is wrong, and even then, as I sat staring at a mental healthcare provider, I resisted the very notion that my problem had anything to do with me.

The therapist seemed to sense that I was conflicted. She smiled and tilted her head, saying, "I'm going to order some blood tests to make sure your body is functioning okay. And then I'm going to refer you to the clinic downtown, because I think your case is outside our range."

"Excuse me?" I said, immediately perking up. I was sure I'd heard her wrong, I *must* have heard her wrong. I had just poured out all my ugliness to this woman and all she had to say was, "I can't help you, here." I was comfortable on campus. I'd spent the better part of five years here. No part of me wanted to venture downtown to a clinic I'd never been to. I felt too raw and exposed, too naked and far too real.

She held up one hand, weighted down with silver bracelets and rings, "you can continue to see me until you graduate, if you think that will help." I chewed on my lip and looked past her, at a fake orchid that sat in the corner of her office. I was set to graduate with my master's degree in a couple of months. I wasn't sure I had it in me to continue seeing her. After our one session, I felt as if I'd been awake for days, my mind as exhausted as my body.

When I emerged from the office, Chad was waiting. "I thought it would be an hour," he said.

"How long was it?" I replied, blinking up at him. Turns out, I'd been sitting in the office with the kind therapist who wore a floral skirt for nearly two and a half hours. "Thank you for waiting," I said, but for some reason, I wasn't feeling grateful. I was just tired, a little annoyed, and empty.

That was the beginning of my recovery, although I didn't know it at the time. What lay ahead was hard: countless therapy sessions, dietitians, Eating Disorder Anonymous (EDA) meetings, and difficult conversations with more than one doctor.

People talk about hitting rock bottom, and I thought my meeting with the therapist was it. But just about a week later, my real bottom came, when I worked up the courage to go to the clinic downtown. I was poked and prodded by a nurse, who glanced down at my blood test results before leaving me alone in a white, sterile room wearing a blue paper gown over my bra and underwear. I kicked my feet. Cracked my neck. Waited impatiently until a tall doctor walked in. He had nice shoes, I noticed. Real leather. He picked up a stool and put it down next to me, so we were almost eye level.

"I hear you're having some problems," he said.

I nodded.

"Well, I need to tell you that your liver enzymes, particularly two called AST and ALT, are very high. What this means is that you're putting a lot of stress on your body. Your heart rate also seems accelerated and," he paused, "I don't think you're well." He waited

to see if I had anything to offer.
I didn't.

"Sarah, can I be very frank with you?"

I nodded again, letting my gaze linger around the small room. I wanted to look anywhere but directly at him.

"There are two things you can do right now. You can choose to get help and get better. *Or* you can choose to continue what you're doing, and you will eventually die. It might not be for a long time, but that's a very real possibility" He looked very tired, and I felt my heart race, my face flushing with shame. "I've seen so many women and men pass through these doors and not live to see their next birthday," he said. "I don't want that to happen to you."

I wished the ground would open and swallow me whole, spitting me out anywhere but in this tiny room with a kind doctor who seemed to genuinely care about me. I wasn't used to people being so forthright. I was used to hiding and avoiding being noticed. My back started sweating.

"I'm going to have the nurse set you up with a care team and you can discuss a treatment plan. Is that alright with you?" he finished.

I nodded for a third time, my tongue dry and heavy in my mouth.

I never intended to harm myself, or maybe I did. I knew that being smaller meant I could run faster, but somewhere along the way, being small became the only thing that mattered. I was taking drastic measures to lose weight, not thinking that my actions were directly affecting my body. Most of the time I didn't feel comfortable in my body at all. I *did* want to get better. I *did* want to stop hating my body and hurting my body and crying into toilets, but I was scared. I was terrified that if I let go of this eating disorder, I wouldn't know who I was anymore. My short visit with that doctor was the real turning point, and my first step on a very long road to recovery.

***

Over two years later, I sat in a circle of chairs in a dingy, one-story building in Newport Beach, CA where Chad and I moved together a year after graduation. When I walked through the door, all I saw were a few plastic chairs set up around a card table. A few people milled about, and I plopped myself down on a chair, conspicuously far from anyone on either side of me. A local Eating Disorders Anonymous (EDA) group rented this room once a week for their meetings. It was only the second meeting I had been to, and I was feeling good about how far I'd come in recovery. I had gotten through the first steps of my treatment plan: I was eating regularly, my body weight was stabilized, and I'd seen two different therapists. I'd read books about recovery, and all my blood tests showed positive improvements.

Many of my early therapy sessions run together in my brain. I cried a lot, and got angry, and continued to battle bouts of restriction and purging. Purging was something I did when my life felt out of control or chaotic, and finding new ways to cope was uncomfortable, like a tag that scratches your neck even after you rip it off. I started writing more, going for long walks, and painting to keep my hands and mind occupied. Nothing I painted was any good, but it seemed to help. Therapy itself was weird and eye-opening, like looking at myself in a funhouse mirror. I recognized myself most of the time, but sometimes my inner world still shocked me in its depth and culpability.

One therapist had me write notes to people that I never sent: my parents, my grandparents, my coaches, my teammates, my boyfriend. I never sent them because I was too embarrassed, and because most people in my life had no idea that I was even seeing a therapist in the first place. Most people had no idea how often I threw up or how much time I spent dreaming about food as I simultaneously restricted myself, and admitting to these trespasses felt silly and juvenile. So what if I threw up every now and then when there were people with much greater problems, suffering far worse than I ever did. My therapist called this "emotional invalidation," and urged me to take ownership of my problems.

"I don't *want* these problems though," I remember telling her.

"You can't heal a cut that you keep reopening," she said.

She also suggested I try a group setting and I agreed because I was lonely. I was gainfully employed by this time, and when the meeting leader passed a basket around at the beginning of the meeting, I watched people plop change into it. A few people threw in one-dollar bills. When the basket came to me, the only bill I could dig up was a five, so I dropped it in. The collection basket helped pay for the meeting space, or so they said. When I dropped the five-dollar bill in the basket, a girl next to me raised her eyebrows. "Sheesh," she said. "Someone came with *cash* today." I felt my face flush even though I had nothing to be embarrassed about.

The meeting proceeded as usual; we all said the EDA prayer. We took turns talking about the topic of the week, which was making reparations. I didn't have much to say because I hadn't made reparations. I barely talked about my eating disorder at all, to anyone. Person after person spoke about apologizing to their loved ones, not for the pain they had themselves endured, but for the pain their eating disorder had caused. Person after person told worse and wilder stories, *See how bad I was?* they seemed to be saying. *I was mean to my mom, I hid things from my family, I terrorized my boyfriend, I lost all my friends.* It was as if we were all competing to see who was the most fucked up and I remember thinking, "I don't belong here. These people *really* need help." Of course, I also needed help, which is why I was there in the first place.

The meeting ended up having the perverse effect of making me feel like I wasn't sick "enough." We all want to have the most sensational story, the most intense rock bottom, the most severe fall from grace. We want to be the best at being at our worst, and my bottom seemed to be the top for some of these people. I found myself wondering if I had a problem at all.

My rational brain knew that I *did* have a problem. I spent a lot of my life telling myself that my eating disorder wasn't real because it wasn't bad enough. People are still denied treatment because their healthcare providers don't categorize them as "sick enough," which usually means, not thin enough, and not close enough to death to warrant intervention.

Our healthcare system is broken in many ways, but perhaps in no way so obviously as when it comes to mental health. I could have sought help earlier, before my body weight dipped too low or my hair started thinning or my liver started shutting down. But I probably would have been turned away, my insurance claims denied, because on the outside, I didn't *look* like I had a problem. I just looked a little thin, a little bony, a little mousey, a little quiet.

After the meeting, the girl who leered at my five-dollar bill approached me and asked, "this your first meeting?"

"It's my first meeting *here*," I emphasized.

She didn't seem to care. Her hair was cut short, and she was covered in tattoos. Her lips were dry, I noticed, and her eyes never looked directly into mine.

"Have you ever gone to a narc abuse support group?" she asked.

I shook my head, not really knowing what she meant.

"My mom was such a narcissist, she really fucked me up. Even now, she's always fishing for compliments, always cutting me down. But this support group gets *deep*, it's *way* better than this one," she said, gesturing backward over her shoulder toward the building we'd just exited. "Let me know if you want to go sometime." I nodded and started walking toward my car, her following in my footsteps.

"Thanks, I will," I said as I unlocked my car door, sliding inside the driver's seat and closing the door firmly behind me. She stood on the sidewalk staring into my car, and my eyes happened to be level with her torso. I noticed dozens of scars lining her forearms. Maybe she was on something, I thought, or lots of things. Eating disorders are addictions, and it isn't uncommon for people to suffer from multiple disorders all at once: depression, anxiety, alcoholism, drug abuse. I was suddenly very aware that the world can be ugly and cruel in ways I hadn't yet imagined. I rolled down my window and smiled up at her. "Really, thank you," I said, "I'd love to check it out." I took a slip of paper she was offering me, that had her name and number scrawled on it in hard, pointy writing. I started up my clunky Ford Taurus and drove home. I never saw her again, and I never went back to another EDA meeting.

LET'S TALK ABOUT MENSTRUATION

During my time as a high school athlete, I was recruited by dozens of collegiate cross country and track programs, mostly from the Midwest with some scattered interest from coaches in Texas, Tennessee, and Ohio. The colleges who were seriously recruiting me were not already winning championships. They were either rebuilding their programs or content with middle of the road performances. Nonetheless, the attention I received from schools and coaches felt validating and somewhat baffling. Navigating the world of collegiate recruiting placed my future almost entirely in my own hands in a way that was both heady and uncomfortable. As I talked with different coaches, I learned to distinguish truth from a good story. The bits of naivety that still clung to me like delicate spiderwebs drifted away as I came to understand who I could trust, and how.

One sunny autumn afternoon after cross country practice, I received a call from the coach at the University of Texas A&M at Corpus Christi. After the obligatory inquiries about my latest races and schoolwork, he got down to business.

"I have to ask you," he said, "if your menstrual cycle is regular? I've found that many of our girls lose their cycle and it's a precursor to injury. We take measures to ensure our team stays healthy so they can perform their best."

How awkward, I thought, before answering, "Actually my period isn't regular at all. I've only had it once." I figured I may as well be honest. I wasn't bothered by my lack of menstruation and was somewhat relieved to avoid that messy element of womanhood.

"Ahhh," he murmured, "thank you for telling me. I need you to understand that if you choose to come run for me, this will be taken seriously. My girls all meet with the team doctor and we can usually get things normalized through proper nutrition and supplementation."

I was stymied. Of the dozens of coaches I spoke with, the Texas A&M at Corpus Christi coach was the only one who brought up menstruation. He drew a parallel between running, eating disorders, menstruation, and injury that was entirely uncomfortable for 17-year-old me, likely because it struck so close to home.

Eating disorders are not uncommon in the running community. A 2018 report in the Journal of Clinical Sports Psychology found that up to 45 percent of female athletes and 19 percent of male athletes struggle with an eating disorder.[1]

The Texas A&M at Corpus Christi coach wanted to discuss my menstrual cycle because he knew that elite runners can easily fall into the pit of disordered eating. He also knew that being lighter did not necessarily mean being faster, especially if being lighter meant starvation and injury. Lack of a regular period is one sign of the female athlete triad, which is only a small part of RED-S.

RED-S stands for "relative energy deficiency in sport"[2] and is the result of insufficient caloric intake and/or excessive energy output. People with eating disorders, especially athletes, often suffer from both. RED-S can alter many physiological systems, including metabolism, menstrual function, bone health, immunity, protein synthesis, and cardiovascular and psychological health.

The RED-S concept was adapted from the female athlete triad, which affects active women with low-energy availability, menstrual dysfunction, and low bone mineral density. I didn't know about the female athlete triad until late in my college career, when a big, fat light bulb went off in my head and I thought, *that's what my problem is.* I didn't learn about RED-S until I was halfway through my master's degree and seeing a therapist for my

---

1   Donna Raskin, "How Athletes Can Navigate Disordered Eating Habits," Runner's World, March 3, 2023, https://www.runnersworld.com/nutrition-weight-loss/a43165676/disordered-eating/
2   Elissa Rosen, MD, CEDS, "RED-S: A More Comprehensive Term for the Effects of Low Energy Intake in Athletes," Gaudiani Clinic, April 1, 2018, https://www.gaudianiclinic.com/gaudiani-clinic-blog/2018/8/1/red-s-a-more-comprehensive-term-for-the-effects-of-low-energy-intake-in-athletes

eating disorder. My first therapist was the one who introduced the concept of RED-S and ordered that my liver enzymes be checked via a blood test. When the results came back, she called me. "Losing your period is only one small part of RED-S," she said, "You might be chronically fatigued, have a lot of, shall we say, gastrointestinal *distress*, and you're likely disrupting your metabolism and a bunch of hormones. That's why your liver enzymes tested so high. I would love to get your hormones tested as well, but I'll have to refer you out for that."

She was right on all accounts. I *was* chronically fatigued, my nails peeled and broke, my hair was thin, and I couldn't run more than a couple of miles without desperately searching for a restroom. High liver enzymes (specifically the enzymes ALT and AST) have been shown to be elevated in cases of chronic starvation. High liver enzymes can also be caused by things like alcoholism, hepatitis, diabetes, certain cancers, and a bunch of other factors. They are not definitive markers of RED-S or of an eating disorder and need to be considered alongside a variety of other factors; in my case, not eating was a glaring one. [3]

For most of my life, I associated losing my menstrual cycle with fitness and felt a real sense of failure when I did occasionally bleed. This attitude was underscored by the mentality of those around me, specifically, my coaches and team doctors who validated and normalized the loss of menstruation. "It's just because you're so fit," they told me each autumn during my yearly physical, "it's nothing serious."

Menstruation is not a cozy, comfortable subject to discuss over dinner, and growing up, I hated the idea of dealing with a monthly cycle. My first period came when I was thirteen and didn't come back until my senior year. For nearly five years, I had only two periods. The first time I tried to use a tampon, I couldn't figure out where to put it and turned to Google for step-by-step

---

[3] Karajibani M, Montazerifar F, Hosseini R, Suni F, Dashipour A R, et al. The Relationship Between Malnutrition and Liver Enzymes in Hospitalized Children in Zahedan: A Case-control Study.Zahedan J Res Med Sci.2021;23(1):e102994.https://doi.org/10.5812/zjrms.102994.

instructions on how to locate my vagina and where to insert a tampon. The fact that I found periods so horrifying and confusing speaks volumes about how I was taught to conceptualize not only my own body, but women's bodies in general. Periods were not something anyone talked about, which is another reason my discussion with the Texas A&M coach was uncomfortable. Every other coach was speaking my language — how to be fast, and how to be skinny. The Texas coach was talking about health and longevity, and I listened, but I simply wasn't interested.

The belief that being thinner results in better athletic performance is still fed to athletes everywhere. To some degree, it is true that lighter bodies can move more quickly through space. It is also important that I underscore that lightness = speed is only true, *to a point*. The problem that so many athletes and coaches overlook is that every body is different. My lightest weight could be another girl's heaviest, and we could still both be strong, fast, and healthy. There is no one-size-fits all formula when it comes to weight: gaining it, losing it, maintaining it, or maybe if you're lucky, forgetting about it entirely.

THE ADULTS IN THE ROOM

"Bradley keeps calling me, asking for money," I tell my parents, during one of our weekly phone calls. I'm chopping vegetables for a salad, my phone in my Grand Canyon sweatshirt pocket and Bluetooth headphones in my ears. "They were good to you," my dad says, "maybe someday, you'll be able to pay it forward."

I attended Bradley University on a full scholarship from 2011 to 2016. My scholarship was part athletic and part academic, which I always point out to underscore that I didn't get to go to college for free just because I was a jock. I had some smarts, or at least, I was smart enough to memorize everything I needed to know before a test, only to forget it soon after.

When I was growing up, my family didn't have a lot of extra money. I was not from the wealthy, upper middle-class suburbs of Chicago like a lot of kids who went to Bradley. There were no private tutors, expensive tennis lessons, or summer vacations. Comparison is the thief of joy, but comparison is also revealing. You never know how much you have until it's taken away, and you never know how little you have until you see how much someone else possesses.

Bradley is not only a private university, but it's also a nonprofit, and in fiscal year 2022, Bradley held a $341 million endowment, according to the National Association of College and University Business Officers. Per tax documents, the university operated in the black for most of fiscal year 2012 through fiscal year 2022.[4] Recently, the school announced that it would be cutting over 20 programs and eliminating 68 faculty positions due to budget shortfalls and the violation of a bond covenant. The more you have, the more it hurts to lose.

At any rate, when my father says that someday, I'll be in a

---

4   Natalie Schwartz, "Bradley University looks to cut over 20 programs and 68 faculty positions," Higher Ed Dive, November 8, 2023, https://www.highereddive.com/news/bradley-university-program-faculty-cuts/699085/

financial position to "pay it forward," I always reply, "Sure, after I make millions." Because if I'm going to donate money to a cause, it's sure as hell not going to wow anyone in terms of zeros, and it's sure as hell not going to a university that charges students more than $50,000 each year to attend. When I attended Bradley, tuition was closer to $40,000, and I know what you might be thinking. You might be thinking, "Wow! You received a $200,000 education and didn't have to pay a dime!" You might also be thinking, "What did you end up doing with such an illustrious, expensive degree?"

You might then find it funny that my first job out of college paid me an annual salary of $35,000. I was working as a grant writer for a housing nonprofit in the south side of Chicago, with all the adult accoutrement like benefits and a retirement plan. But $35,000 didn't leave a lot left over at the end of each month, so to make ends meet, I moonlighted as a babysitter for young families in the suburbs of Chicago, where I routinely made hundreds of dollars in cash for a day or two of childcare. My degrees were fine and all, but they had nothing to do with the crispy $100 bills that paid for rent and groceries.

When I first visited Bradley, I was introduced to a couple of staff members in the English Department. Dr. Lee, who would eventually become one of my academic advisors, and Shelly, the English Department secretary, who sat in a cozy office decorated to look like a Thomas Kinkade painting, where students hung out before, after, and in between classes so Shelly could never get any blessed work done. They were nice, but at the time of my visit, I never once thought, *I'll see them again.*

Fast forward a few years and I'm sitting in one of Dr. Lee's classes. We're talking about how difficult it is for people who immigrate to America to feel at home in their new country, full of new laws, new customs, new people, and new languages. "Some of you might feel a similar way," Dr. Lee said, "though of course to a lesser degree. Going away to college can often leave young adults feeling untethered and alone. There may be customs, laws, people, even language that is new and uncomfortable to you."

Yes, I thought, and my mind flashed to memories of family dinners back home. My father, sitting at our kitchen table after supper, tipping back in his chair and saying (of his boss), "he thinks his own *shit* don't *stink*." I thought of our family reunions, my aunts and uncles standing outside a white paneled garage to smoke cigarettes. I thought of my high school freshman English class, when a boy who read at a third-grade level was called on to read the part of Romeo, whose life never gave him a shot at academic success. I thought of leaving home while my mother was still undergoing cancer treatments, the guilt I felt over leaving, the way everything about my life felt untethered and not real.

School was my one saving grace because classrooms were predictable; I knew how to play the academic game. Succeeding in school was simply a matter of following a set of pre-established rules, but even as I pulled straight A's, I felt conflicted about my decision to leave home. Part of me felt like I'd abandoned myself by pursuing a private education, and a degree in English no less. What good did writing do, when the summer was so dry that all the corn turned to brown ash? What good did it do to tell a compelling story, when sickness and economic insecurity were clawing at the edges of home? What good did it do to embrace my past when it was so radically different, even diametrically opposed, to the future I was facing?

For the most part, I didn't fit in at this private university that was overflowing with money, connections, and prestige. Some of my classmates went to Europe over winter break. Some studied abroad. Some were in expensive sororities or lived in the brand new off-campus housing that I knew for a fact didn't have decades old carpet stains or smell slightly of mildew. I spent holidays working and taking classes, always running, always training, and always tired. My clothing came from TJ Maxx and thrift stores, before thrift stores were posh and cool. Sometimes when I stood in line at the grocery store, I'd covertly check my banking app to confirm I had enough cash. Based on the number, I'd stay in line or slip away to put a few items back. All of this felt huge, but it wasn't. Not feeling like I belonged was the one thing that held me back the most.

The summer before I completed my masters, I was visiting home and attended a church service with my mother. The county sheriff was part of our parish, and he asked what I was doing with my life.

"Getting my Masters degree," I answered.

He was retired at this point, his large, bowling belly hanging heavily over his starched Sunday pants. His mustache had turned gray, and his eyebrows rose slightly at my answer. "Don't be getting too smart for us now," he said, his voice joking, but his eyes serious.

I was smart enough to know when to remain silent. I went back to Bradley and tried to imagine what someone like me, with an M.A. in English, would do for work if I moved back home. I thought about it for the entirety of my seven-hour drive back to campus and for the life of me, I couldn't find an answer.

My father still believes that someday, I'll be able to make a large donation to Bradley University. "You'd better get to working on that bestselling novel," he'll say, and I don't have the heart to tell him that I've never written a believable bit of fiction, that I'm only a half-good writer anyway, and that most writers don't get rich. His insistence that I'm good at what I do is often the only reason I believe it. My father is not a man to mince words, and prides himself on saying exactly what he thinks. Candor was something I sorely missed as I navigated the new customs and language of a university, where I learned that the truth is not always obvious, fiction can look a hell of a lot like fact, and the adults in the room are often just as confused as any kid.

HEY, COACH

Coaches are vital to athlete development, especially for young adult athletes. I was lucky to have terrific coaches when I was a kid, from the time I started running in sixth grade all the way up to my high school graduation. The reason my coaches were so great is because I was coached mostly by the same person: a man named Joe Doucette who everyone called coach D. He was a smart coach, knowing when to push us and knowing when to hit the brakes. I was always eager to do more, and he recognized that, if left to my own devices, I would run myself ragged.

When I went on to compete collegiately, I had to adjust to a very different coaching style. My coaches were old school, and collegiate coaching was, and still is, heavily male in a way that felt a bit like a fraternity. All the coaches from any school we competed against seemed to know one another. Like any business, the more a coach networked the quicker he could climb the ladder to a coaching job at a large school with a bigger budget and a higher salary. My high school coach cared about my wellbeing because he was a good person and his livelihood did not depend on my performance. All Coach D wanted was for his athletes to grow and do well.

My college coaches came to Bradley to build a small, average team into national champions. We were bodies to them, numbers in a formula designed to launch their coaching careers. I was motivated and naïve enough to believe everything they told me, so when they told me to lose weight, I did. And then, because they tied performance to the size of our bodies so heavily and so often, I lost more. I knew more about my own body than they ever could, but for some reason, I chose to listen to them.

At the time, NIL (name, image, and likeness) deals did not exist, and college athletes could not be legally compensated by any outside sponsors or organizations. I couldn't accept prize money at a local 4th of July 10k, and I couldn't (again, legally) receive compensation when the school used my name and image on marketing materials. My compensation was my scholarship, and the coaches were the ones who decided how to spread the available scholarship aid. To their credit, they did not revoke scholarships for poor performances or injuries. But they did decide who got to compete and when. They dictated our financial aid, our daily schedules, and a large chunk of our time. Even if I'd wanted to walk away, my scholarship and therefore, my future livelihood, felt at stake.

Collegiate athletics is a system that is built not around athlete well-being, health, or even long-term success, but rather around short-term success so that the people in charge can get paid. For myself and for the women I trained alongside, the people in positions of power were men. During formative years of our lives, their coaching tactics put our long-term health at-risk. The culture of collegiate athletics was broken, and in buying into a broken system, I unwittingly broke myself.

The men who coached me didn't know much about how women's bodies develop or perform. They trained us as if we were small men, normalizing the absence of menstrual cycles and pushing us to be smaller until our smallness made us weak. They "inspired" us by shaming us, and praised and perpetuated disordered behavior. It was an abusive and detrimental dynamic that many of us didn't come to fully understand until we were out of the collegiate system.

My coaches, like many coaches, placed undue emphasis on our weight. They weighed us weekly and checked our body fat with calipers in the weight room, in front of everyone. My roommate went home one summer and came back to campus emaciated because our coaches told her she'd be faster if she shed a few pounds from her already thin frame. After I voiced my concern, my coaches pulled me aside and told me that her starvation was really *dedication* and that runners need to *look different* to perform well. They told me I should take the hint and maybe I'd be faster, too. So, I lost 10, 15, 20, 25 pounds, and they praised me for how *fit* I looked. They blamed my poor races or training sessions on weight instead of examining a multitude of other, more realistic, factors.

My Sophomore year, I was nominated for a campus-wide "Athlete of the Year" award and didn't win, the award going instead to a woman from the golf team. She was an accomplished athlete who deserved the recognition, but my coaches were enraged.

"She doesn't even *look* like an athlete," one of them spat, spinning in his high-backed office chair. "She's *disgusting*."

I cringed at their words but remained silent because I had too much invested in my team, my sport, and these coaches to give up my belief in what they told me.

Many of my teammates have since bonded over our shared experiences. Our bodies were under a microscope, while the men's team seemed largely free of this particular hostility. One of my teammates later pointed out that the behavior of our coaches may seem minor in isolation but the accumulation of them was intensely damaging.

My coaches were not the only coaches engaging in this behavior, and the problem wasn't as shallow as body shaming or gaslighting, though those are both valid. The problem was that these coaches had real power over us. They could take away scholarships. They could exclude us from competition. They could control our time to such a degree that we had little space for anything else.

My attitude toward food before I went to Bradley was already fractured. There is no saying what might have happened if I'd been under different tutelage, or if I'd known what I know now: that being lighter only works to a point, and that no sport is worth killing yourself over.

In 2020, a group of women from the University of Alabama Birmingham came forward with similar complaints about one of their coaches, who was the assistant coach at Bradley for four of my five years there. I published an article in support of them, detailing the many ways his coaching practices harmed not only myself, but so many of my teammates. Most of the feedback I received from that article was positive, but some was very negative. Some people accused me of trying to ruin my old coaches, but that was not possible. There were too many other voices already speaking out, and besides, I was telling the truth.

Truth is an uncomplicated and burning thing, and one of the hardest truths about my experience is that I was actively complicit, actively silent, and easily swayed by their influence. I wanted them to be right so badly that I didn't listen to my own gut instinct. Despite how it seared, I found the truth impossible to face until I was all alone, and very quiet.

***

Years after I graduated from Bradley, I'm home for my brother's wedding. I'm sitting outside with my parents, watching the late afternoon turn into dusk. I forget how long the days are up north, and sat relishing the late evening sun, the sound of tree frogs humming in the swamp, the earth a deep emerald green, and the air sweet with the unmistakable smell of summer. I'm filling my parents in on everything that happened after graduation, the drama with the University of Alabama Birmingham athletes, and what I know of my old coaches.

"One of them is selling treadmills now," I tell my father, "And the other," I pause, looking down the road toward our neighbors' red barn glowing in the late evening light, "I'm not sure what he's doing. I think he's coaching at a private high school somewhere."

My father thinks for a moment before answering, careful to toe the delicate line between support for me, his only daughter, and the natural empathy men extend to one another.

"Well," he says, "I hope they're both doing okay now. I always thought, you know," he paused to sigh, crossing his large arms over his chest, "that they were both *okay*. I thought they were doing their best and it's just…" he looks at me over his glasses, "maybe they deserve a second chance."

I let silence hang for a moment, and it grows heavier as I hold my tongue. "They were awful," I spit, unable to contain my frustration. My mind wanders back to me hobbling around a track with a bum hip, limping around campus on crutches, sitting in a hospital room with a kind doctor who told me that if I didn't change, my path would end in an early death.

My father stares down the road, and I stare at my feet, my toenail polish gleaming white against the dark earth. In my heart, I know my father is right. Holding onto this anger will hurt nobody but myself. I sigh heavily, digging my toes further into the dirt, and let the words fall out, "Maybe they do. I just *really, really* hope they've changed."

My eyes drift down the road to where my father is still gazing, at a bridge marked with yellow and black striped signs. The bridge only covers a small creek that runs dry in the summer and overflows in the spring. I love the bridge because it always felt like it was mine, like it held secrets nobody else could possibly understand. When I was young, I'd hang over its edge and watch the water flow by, wondering what might lie beneath its surface. I repeat myself, because that's what my father does, so that's what I do, too. "I just really hope they've changed."

BAD BOYFRIEND

Chad was the boyfriend that every girl has once; the boyfriend you love precisely because you know you should not. He was the boyfriend who constantly gave me butterflies, which I took as a sign of severe attraction. I didn't learn until years later that butterflies are more often a sign of anxiety and stress, and my relationship with Chad had resentment growing at its very center. Would he text me back? Would his message be flirty or indifferent? Would he ignore me in front of his friends and then punch a wall when I chatted up one of his closest buddies? Women everywhere have known a Chad, or a version of him; a guy who adores you to the point of disgust before sticking his teeth in your neck to suck out any ounce of self-respect.

Before dating Chad, I dated a boy in the ROTC program who was kind and smart and made me laugh. ROTC boy was everything I should have wanted and nothing I did. He was a farm boy and a true gentleman, totally devoid of deception and malice. I traded loyalty for uncertainty, and honesty for false charm.

Chad and I both ran cross country and track, and our lives paralleled in a way that I thought made sense. I was running upwards of 70-miles a week, and he was hitting 90-100. We ran together, worked, lifted weights, and generally lived and breathed our sport. Chad was a fast runner, with a tall gangly frame that made me feel hugely muscular yet tiny at the same time. Like me, Chad didn't grow up with much money. He delivered papers throughout high school, dragging himself out of bed every day at 4 a.m. to sling local news out a car window. His work ethic was fanatical, and I quietly admired his hustle. Together we worked, ran, studied, worked, ran, studied. I studied more than he did, and he worked more than me. I fell hard for his baby blue eyes and long blonde hair that tumbled in perfect soft spiral curls. I loved how easily we fell into rhythm and how, at the start, he showered me with attention and gifts. We didn't know it, or couldn't see it, but our partnership was doomed to combust.

Chad and I were together nearly two years when I heard that he'd been talking to other girls. The newness of the relationship had melted away by then, and our inner lives crept closer to the surface. He was uncovering insecurity, and I was uncovering emotional unavailability. I was a slave to my eating disorder, and I couldn't make enough room in my brain to care about it and him both. Something had to give. So, when I found out that he had been talking to other girls, I assumed it was my fault. I hadn't been available enough. I hadn't given him enough sex. I hadn't been exotic enough. I had become mundane, leading him to seek excitement elsewhere. If he had just been flirting, I might have forgiven him, but he had been offering much more than flirtation. He'd also been offering sex, and with it, pictures of his body. I have yet to meet a woman who truly enjoys receiving a dick pic, yet there are so many men craning their necks and sharply bending their elbows and flexing their abs, all so that someone can look at their privates with utter indifference at best.

I found out more about Chad's inner life one summer I was home visiting my family before the cross-country season was set to start. I received a Facebook message from a stranger:

> *Hey sorry if this is weird,* she wrote, *but are you Chad's girlfriend?*
>
> *Yeah,* I answered, *Why?*

And she sent me half a dozen screenshots in quick succession. They started flirtatious and ended overtly sexual.

I didn't sleep for two days straight, vacillating between choking on white hot anger and a fat caterpillar of shame. "Have you ever had a reason not to trust dad?" I asked my mother the morning after the Facebook messages. We were standing in the kitchen next to the trash can, my eyes hollow and drooping.

"Honey, *never.* I trust your father completely," she answered, pulling me into a tight embrace. In the sober light of day, standing in my childhood home, my anger and sadness seemed almost absurd. I had so much love here, why was I looking for it anywhere else?

I drove the seven hours back to Peoria planning what I would say to Chad. He knew that I knew about his indiscretions, and I thought about all the different ways I could hurt him back. *An eye for an eye, and the whole world is blind.* But when I barged through the door, all I could ask was, *How could you?* Showering him with the one question he didn't have a good answer to: *why?*

We had moved in together by then, our lives intermingling in such stupid finite ways that separating seemed extra painful. Our laundry tossed together in the hamper, his dishes beside mine in the cupboard. Our low-budget college apartment was cramped and old but homey. Looking around at it then, it seemed foreign and hostile.

Chad was on his feet, his arms clasped in front of him, pleading, "I didn't mean it, I was never going to do anything, I don't even *know* her. Sarah, I *love* you. I'm so sorry, I was drunk, and I fucked up."

Before that day, I believed that he loved me because he *said* he loved me, and I'd never had reason to doubt anybody's love before. "I just need some space," I said, locking myself in our bedroom with the cat. Chad slept on the couch for a week before I allowed him back into the room.

It was inevitable that we would fall back together, our unique traumas and insecurities pushing us into each other's orbit. He promised to change, and I held on tight to how he was in the beginning, sweet and attentive and devastatingly charismatic. Chad wanted us to move on and forget about what he'd done. He apologized, but I couldn't help holding onto a shard of resentment and anger that stuck sorely in my side and caused me to mistrust everything he did and every word he said.

At the end of the school year, I had my M.A. degree and Chad had his Bachelors. I landed a job working at a nonprofit in the South Side of Chicago, and we moved there together. He picked up a job at a local running store before being offered full-time employment working for a shoe company. When winter set in, we booked a trip to Colorado where he proposed to me on the side of a mountain. I said yes, because that's what you do when you're 23 and your boyfriend is on bended knee. We never talked about getting married, and I'd never been one to imagine myself white-veiled and dewy-skinned and desperately in love. I think I understood, even then, that love was never so simple. A year after we moved to Chicago, Chad had the opportunity to transfer to Southern California for the same role in a new territory. I agreed to go, hoping that a change in location might make us truly happy again.

We had flown to California for track meets before, racing under the lights at Stanford and traveling to Long Beach and Azusa Pacific. In the dead of Illinois winter, California was bright and stunningly beautiful. My pale skin turned pink in the sun and when we visited the ocean, we ran into the water, shocked at how cold it was. I loved California but I never imagined I'd live there. So, when we made the long drive from Illinois to Orange County, I felt like I'd been living in the dark and was only just beginning to understand light.

As we settled into our new life in Southern California, I realized the grave error I'd made in assuming a new place would change us in any meaningful way. Suddenly apart from anyone and everything we knew, we leaned so hard on each other that we eventually gave way, like an overloaded tension bridge. I attempted to make new friends, and Chad grew jealous of anyone new that I spent time with. He was traveling a lot for his job and drank heavily when he was home. I relished the nights spent without him and dreaded his return the same way you might dread a root canal. When he was home, my stress increased tenfold. We fought constantly and his unpredictable moods set me on edge. I found myself tip toeing on eggshells: one wrong word, and he'd explode. Meanwhile, the burden of planning our wedding fell squarely on my shoulders. I flew home to Wisconsin, where I half-heartedly bought a dress on clearance at David's Bridal. My mom and grandmother went with me, taking turns picking out dresses and critiquing which ones fit my body best. We found a wedding venue near my family, and as the big day grew closer, I dragged my feet on sending out the invites. I had sent out the obligatory "Will you be my bridesmaid?" cards, but the wedding invitations sat neatly on our desk. Messages from his family and mine all carried the same tone: *When is the wedding? Where is my invitation? Shouldn't you send out a save the date?* It was supposed to be a late spring wedding, pinks, and greens with ruby red accents. My dress was sleeveless and simple. I planned to wear my mother's wedding veil.

One night, shortly before Halloween and only eight months before our wedding date, Chad and I dressed up as Pooh Bear (me) and Christopher Robin (him) and went to a party hosted by one of the higher ups at his company.

The party host was a man in his late sixties who worked because he wanted to, not because he had to. The party was at his expansive home that overlooked a rolling green canyon. He hired a private caterer who continually offered us decadent appetizers, which we declined because we were, at that time, both vegan. There was an open bar with a specially made cocktail that Chad drank so many of I eventually lost track, the alcohol hitting his empty stomach hard and fast. Within a couple of hours, his mood was spiraling out of control, and I felt myself grow small in the tall shadow of alcohol.

As the party was winding down, I went to find the bathroom. When I came back, he was outside on their stone patio smoking a joint and he offered it to me.

"Come on," he said, laughing, his blue eyes, the same eyes I'd fallen in love with nearly five years earlier, danced with danger. "Try some."

"I'm good," I said, not knowing how my body would react to weed. I never smoked, and not only did I not know how my body would react, I wanted to stay in control of my body and my emotions. My refusal of the joint sparked a flash of anger.

"Well, what *do* you want?" he snapped, his voice rising. I looked around at the ever-thinning crowd and answered quietly, "I think I want to go home."

This small request set him into a fury. Recognizing an angry outburst about to happen, I quickly thanked the hosts and made an exit, pushing through the wide glass front door, past the manicured lawn, and into the quiet street. We hadn't walked more than a few dozen feet when he started yelling at me, "You're *such a bitch!*" he said, "That's my *boss* and you were so fucking *rude*, you're such a goddamned *cunt* sometimes, Sarah."

I started walking faster, toward the exit of the flawless gated community where civilized people lived, people who surely did not scream at each other in the street, people who surely had the decency to yell at each other *inside*, at the very least. I felt small and stupid, like white trash from some seedy part of town. *We don't belong here*, I thought. I couldn't pretend that I fit in here, in an opulent community in one of the wealthiest counties in the nation, with my drunk fiancé making a scene and cold sweat making streaks through my red shirt. I saw a light go on in a window and I picked up the pace, urgently ordering an Uber to take us home.

We sat on a curb as we waited for the Uber, my Pooh-Bear ears tilting crookedly on my head. Chad was on a hot rant, "You don't even want to fucking marry me, you just care about *you*. I don't even know why I bother taking you places, it's so embarrassing, you're seriously such a *cunt*, you know that? Nobody in there even *liked* you."

When the driver arrived, we sat on opposite sides of the backseat, Chad continuing his tirade, me doing my best to hold back tears. When we arrived back at our apartment complex, Chad stormed upstairs and the Uber driver, a short balding man in a neat white button up shirt, turned around and looked at me.

"He seems really upset," he said, eyeing me through wire-rimmed glasses. "Are you okay?" His small nose scrunched up a bit, as if he smelled something putrid.

"I'm fine," I said, my voice sounding small, "He's just like this when he's drunk."

The Uber driver nodded slowly and said, "Well I'll stay here for a few, come outside if you need anything." He was probably a father, I thought, because only a father could care about a strange girl with mascara running down her face and misery shining through her red-rimmed eyes.

We lived on the second floor of a nice apartment complex, with a patio that faced a busy residential street. When we moved in, I was dazzled by how large and nice the apartment was. The unit had its own washer and dryer, two full-sized bathrooms, and a pool with a hot, luxurious jacuzzi. As I went upstairs that night, I diverted my eyes away from one of our neighbors. I wondered how often she heard us fighting. I'd been on edge for months by this point, and when I opened the door, I was unsurprised to find him waiting.

"What the *fuck*, Sarah? Where *were* you just now?" he asked. "God, I really can't take you anywhere, you're such a *whore*."

When I didn't reply, he stepped close, looming over me, so I could smell the alcohol cutting his breath.

"Answer me! Why won't you *answer* me?!"

Angry outbursts were normal when he was drunk. I was used to him picking fights with other boys or getting in yelling matches at bars. I was even used to insults, which were always followed by apologies in the morning, or a bouquet of flowers, or breakfast. But that night, he took a step back, grabbed a book off an end table, and threw it at me. It missed my head by inches, and I momentarily froze. He never hit me. Usually, he directed his anger at other people or other things, punching walls at a frat house, or getting in a fist fight with another boy. But this time, I was his only target.

"If you don't want to be with me then *don't*," he yelled, stepping toward me.

I inched myself away from the front door and toward the master bedroom, which I could lock.

"Are you *scared*?" he said, incredulously.

I didn't want to answer him, but I knew that saying nothing would make him angrier. I dragged my fingers along the wall until I felt the bedroom door frame. I looked up at him and spat, "*No*" as I whirled inside, slamming the door in his face. I pulled a small dresser in front of the door simply because it made me feel better. He pounded on the wall for a while but gave up easily, I presumed, to pass out drunk on the couch.

I lowered myself to the floor, my legs wobbly and my palms wet. I was a little afraid, and *very* angry. As I sat on our beige carpet sobbing, I realized shamefully that I wasn't even angry at Chad, I was angry at myself. And worse yet, he was right. I didn't want to be with him anymore. Despite how sweet I knew he could be and how attentive he once was, he had shown me his true character years ago. I was stupid for hanging on for as long as I had, for moving across the country with him, for believing his countless apologies, and most of all, for not believing that I deserved better.

As I sat crying, our cat crawled toward me from underneath the bed. The cat was Chad's idea; he was living alone our junior year of college and grew lonely. He found the cat on Craigslist, and it didn't take long for us both to fall in love. We named the cat Chub Chub and as I sat alone on the bedroom floor holding him, I thought about how I would end things. Despite the embarrassment I imagined we'd suffer over the broken engagement, I was too tired and too angry to care.

When he sobered up, I would tell Chad to leave. For now, I would shower in scalding water, wait until it grew lukewarm. I'd wrap myself in a large sweater and thick sweatpants and climb into bed with Chub Chub, who sat atop my chest and purred, like he did every night. Only this time, I was more alone than I'd ever been. I clutched my cat like a lifeline and eventually fell asleep.

In the dreary light of morning, Chad did not apologize. He was hungover and chose to ignore me as I padded around the apartment dusting picture frames and putting things away. External order made my internal chaos feel more manageable and less extreme. The following day was Monday, and after work, I sat down on the couch with Chad and told him I absolutely could not marry him. I watched his face turn from annoyance to disbelief to desperation. For once, I wasn't the one crying.

"I'm not giving up on *us*," he said, raising his long arms in mock defeat, "I can't believe you want to throw this all away."

The next day, he left for a 10-day work trip, and I let myself breathe a bit, my body slowly decompressing in his absence. I spent most of those 10 days alone, planning my escape. I couldn't afford the apartment on my own, but I could probably find a roommate. I started looking for a second source of income, applying for waitressing jobs or nannying gigs, running through my budget with a fine-toothed comb. When Chad returned, he said he treated me poorly because of how I treated him. He offered to go to therapy if I would reconsider the breakup, something I'd begged him to do countless times before. The apartment lease was in my name, so when I refused to continue our relationship, he left. He slowly moved his things, packed his bruises in a large black suitcase, and vanished.

***

Half a decade later, I'm visiting my family during Christmas. My brother and his wife have a nine-month-old baby, William Todd. William has a giant head, bright blue eyes, and two baby teeth popping through his bottom gums. We haven't had a new baby in the family in a very long time, and my mother is awash in the glow of new grandmother-hood.

"He can say *dada*, but he can't quite say mama yet," she's explaining, "which I think is normal, *dada* is much easier to say." My mother and I are standing in the kitchen, around the Formica-topped table and scuffed wooden chairs. She's asking me about my then-boyfriend, Mike, "What's Mike up to today?" she says.

"He's probably still in bed with Chub Chub," I say, "can you believe he [Chub Chub] is getting so old? I feel like I've had him forever."

"When did you and Chad get him, exactly?" asks my mother. And I briefly recount the story of how Chub Chub entered our lives; how Chad saw a photo of an orange and white kitty on Craigslist and decided he needed a pet. How we spent an entire Sunday afternoon making a ninety-minute drive that ended on a rural dead-end road, where I was certain I'd be murdered, or worse. Instead, we met a kind couple who rescued Chub Chub, who they called Gus (can you believe it?), after finding him abandoned at a dump. They already had three cats, or they would have kept him for themselves. "He's a bit shy," the woman told us, "But he'll warm up to you quick."

They gave us a litter box, food, and some toys, and just like that, we were the proud new owners of a dumpster cat. I held Chub Chub in my lap on the drive home, and he peed on my jeans. From that moment on, I told my mother, the cat and I shared an iron bond.

My mother's eyes twinkle as she laughs, but she's heard my story more than once. As her laughter dims, she looks at me hard and says, "You know honey, we had no idea that Chad," she looks away, out the large bay window before finishing her thought, "was so awful to you."

"How could you have known, mum?" I say, and I get the distinct impression that I've relieved my mother of some sort of guilt she's been carrying, for not being able to protect me from all terrifying, hateful parts of the world.

We hug, and I look over her shoulder, out the large bay kitchen window where so many people in my family have gathered over the decades. Where so much hurt and love, forgiveness and laughter has been shared. There is no snow this Christmas, and the land outside is muted and barren, the grass a dull gray-brown, and the naked tree branches stretching towards heaven as if they hope, like all of us do, to one day reach it.

YES, YOU CAN

One morning shortly after Chad moved to Portland, I met a friend for a sunrise run around a local trail system. The scent of sagebrush seeped into our skin, and our faces caught the dozens of spider webs that hung softly across the trails.

"My 20's were a decade of such growth," Megan said. "I mean, you go from being a student, still sort of dependent on your parents, to getting your first job and figuring out whatever corporate system you land in. You learn to be independent; you probably have your heart broken a few times; you probably move. So much change happens, alongside so much growth."

She was trying to comfort me, and even though my heart was raw, I appreciated her effort. We chatted about change, and she told me pieces of her story: going to grad school, moving for her first job, dating a guy who she thought would be her forever person, only to have that person tear her heart in two.

"Being single takes some getting used to," she said. "The person you relied on is suddenly not there. It can feel lonely and disarming but," she waved her hand vaguely toward the sky, as if my ex had moved to the clouds instead of to Portland. "You were so unhappy with him. You're going to find that you're better off without him."

Of course, she was right. I loved Chad enough to try to change myself to make him happy, but that was a losing game. Instead of feeling loved and supported, I felt lonely and judged.

When I told him about big ideas I had—to write a book or start a blog, he would shrug away my ambitions as if they weren't important. "You don't have time to write a book," he'd say. Or, "You're always having ideas. Why bother telling me about this if you're not going to do it?" The way he so easily tore apart my dreams and diminished my excitement made me listless and uncommunicative. Instead of sharing my dreams with him,

I started writing them down. Instead of building something together, we were building separate lives. There was one thing that did keep us together though, and that was running.

Before we broke up, I'd travel with him on some of his weekend work trips, helping him set up his tent and the shoes he'd let people test out. Then I'd wander off to explore the trails or find a coffee shop to read in. One of the first races I attended with him was an ultramarathon called Kodiak that ran in a huge loop around a mountain lake in Big Bear, CA. I was enthralled by everyone who was able to run dozens of miles through mountainous terrain, especially as my sea level lungs struggled to breathe in the thin air. After spending so long in the hyper-competitive world of collegiate running, there was something about trail running that sparked my interest. Most people were testing themselves more than racing against anyone else.

"I want to do this next year," I told Chad "Maybe the 50-miler." And he again, diminished this with a shrug and a statement: "This race is too hard for you. You should start with something smaller."

Instead of feeling discouraged, I felt feral rage. Nothing could inspire me more than hearing that I couldn't do something.

After we broke up, I went online and signed up for the Kodiak 50-miler, defiantly hitting the "register now" button and smirking with satisfaction. I drove to Big Bear every weekend to train, unsure of what to expect on race day because I wasn't sure what I was doing. My friend Stephanie offered to crew me, bringing me a change of shoes, and filling my pack at aid stations. On race morning, I was jittery with nerves and sprinted off the start line, only to fade eventually to a third-place finish. Chad was right, the race *was* hard. I didn't hydrate well enough, or eat enough, but I still finished. As I stood on the podium holding a small, carved wooden bear, I couldn't stop smiling. I trained hard, and it paid off. I was surrounded by friends. I did something I never imagined doing. Megan was right, I was better off without him. Not because we weren't right for each other, but because living with someone who doesn't support your dreams is a sad, slow way to die.

GUNS & STUFF

Growing up in rural Wisconsin meant that hunting was something people did, an activity as common as oil changes and just as messy. Hunting requires weapons, and weapons require knowledge and responsibility. When I was eleven and my brother was twelve, my family decided he could accompany my father on the deer hunt, only to watch, not to shoot. To do this legally, my brother had to complete a gun safety class. My father dragged me along because I had nowhere else to be, and when left to my own devices, I did things like microwave hard boiled eggs and bury inconsequential "treasure," like old chapstick and shiny, tumbled rocks, behind the barn where my brother could not find it.

The gun safety course was held in the middle school/high school cafeteria. Our school district had a single building for K-12, and it was not such a long walk from the fourth-grade rooms full of artwork and large laminated maps to the high school, where kids seemed so big and broken and grown.

The cafeteria was full of men with their sons and a few scattered daughters. A man with a large beard and a bowling ball belly stood in the front of the cafeteria, wearing work boots and a red Colfax Vikings Basketball t-shirt. He talked about the dangers of guns, how to properly carry a gun, clean a gun, shoot a gun, and store a gun. The longer he talked, the more bored I became. I kicked my feet, stared at the bearded man, and tried to imagine myself carrying a gun through a snowy forest to shoot deer or pheasants or ducks or geese. I couldn't imagine myself shooting anything. I *liked* deer and pheasants and ducks and geese.

"Hey," my father said, nudging me with his elbow, "*listen*. This is good for you to know, too."

The instructor was telling a story meant to scare us, and it *was* scary. There was a woman going for a walk, the instructor said, who was wearing a white scarf during gun season. A hunter mistook her scarf for the tail of a deer, and her life was over.

His life was too, in every way that mattered. The ground was probably frozen, I thought, shimmering with that crusty frost that crackles when you walk over it. I wondered if the hunter sank to his knees. I wondered if he ran.

My father always had guns, hunting rifles and a 22 locked in a cabinet in our basement. I don't know where he kept the key, and I never tried to find it. Guns were just another household item, as common as dish soap or lighting fixtures. I never actually knew to be afraid of guns until I learned that guns were bad, or that guns were responsible for things like death, school shootings, and violence. Guns are *bad*, people said, guns are *unnecessary*, guns *kill*.

When I moved to California, I was still holding tightly to a vegan lifestyle. I went out of my way to meet other vegans, and one of my best vegan friends was a girl named Christine.

"Come to Veg Fest with me," she texted me one mild summer afternoon. Veg Fest was a vegan food extravaganza, complete with things like vegan chicken waffles, animal adoptions, and photo opportunities with vegan influencers. We chatted as we wove in between booths, dodging people and scoping out what we wanted to eat. At some point, she asked me what it was like to grow up next to a dairy farm.

"Did it smell?" she said, her brown eyes twinkling with mischief.

"Of course it smelled!" I said back, giggling. It especially smelled in the spring when farmers spread manure over their fields. They did this to improve crop production and soil quality, and (I thought) because what else could we possibly do with the enormous piles of manure? Christine and I settled on starting the afternoon with a plate of vegan nachos.

"Did you ever feel bad for eating meat when you were growing up?" she asked, dipping a chip into a bright yellow cup of cashew cheese.

"No," I answered, giving it some thought. "It was just how we lived. And honestly, we ate a lot more venison than beef or anything."

She wrinkled her nose at me, giving me an impish, sideways smile. "What do you mean by *venison*?"

"Deer," I answered, "We ate deer." I saw her eyebrows rise. "It's actually not that weird," I was quick to assure her, "My dad and brother hunted. It's a lot cheaper than buying meat, and healthier." Somehow, I needed to impress upon my friend that eating deer wasn't cruel or bad. I needed her to know that of all the meat I *could* have eaten, venison was the best.

"I can't believe your family killed deer. *Deer*," Christine said, repeating herself, with a hint of disgust.

I shrugged, "That's just how it was."

"Hmmm," she muttered, "I guess every family has their thing."

I smiled and looked away. My family had much worse "things" than eating venison, and it charmed me a bit that she thought hunting deer was some exotic activity. There are millions of deer hunters nationwide; it is by no means a rare activity.

We spent the rest of the afternoon slinking around the food festival, drinking kombucha and splitting a vegan Oreo shake. As the sun set over the bright food tents, white lights began clicking on. A man pedaled by on a unicycle wearing a t-shirt that read "Meat is Murder." My stomach was full, and I was happily tired from chatting and laughing all day. I thought about being home, soaking in a warm bath. Before we left, I hugged Christine and she said, "*I love you.*" I knew she meant it, and I loved her, too.

When I attended that gun safety class with my dad and brother, I learned that guns are not dangerous on their own. They are dangerous when misused, so instead of fearing guns, I learned to fear people, which is a more useful fear to hold since many of the world's traumas have been executed by humans. However, I was beginning to understand that fearing people is often not useful at all. Southern California offered a culture shock that left me feeling odd and quirky and misunderstood. Maybe I was, but then again, maybe not.

Sometimes I still encounter people who think hunting is wildly inhumane, and I'm probably not going to change their minds. Like many people, I've grown accustomed to buying meat from grocery stores that's dyed pink and wrapped in cellophane. It's easy to forget where that meat came from in the first place. Or maybe we'd rather not think about it. The existence of guns is a different conversation entirely from the sport of hunting, a fact that is often muddied in the discourse about gun reform.

"Biden wants to take our guns away!" one of my high school classmates wrote on Facebook one day, a few days after he also alleged that the sanctity of marriage was at risk and that there are only two God-given genders. His post about Biden had over 100 likes and only one angry face. From my beachside bedroom more than a thousand miles away, I sighed tiredly and closed my phone. His anger is not entirely his own. The sentiment he shared is also held by a large portion of the nation, a new manifestation of an older and much deeper divide.

There were some things my new friends in California couldn't quite understand, though, like one of my high school AP Biology projects. We were instructed to either find a dead animal or hunt one, remove the meat from its bones, disassemble the bones, and put the skeleton of the animal back together again. My brother shot a rabbit for me, and a friend and I skinned the rabbit, boiled the meat off its bones, bleached and dried the bones, and slowly glued them back together with Gorilla glue. I did not find the assignment macabre. I found it tedious and even a little pointless.

"Couldn't you just look at a diagram?" Christine asked when I recounted the story to her. I suppose we could have, but then we would not have gone outside, touched the bones, or understood just how delicate this life really is.

DR. T. AND AMY THE DIETITIAN

To the woman he said, 'I will surely multiply your pain in childbearing; in pain you shall bring forth children. Your desire shall be contrary to your husband, but he shall rule over you.'

— *Genesis 3:16*

"There is no greater gift for women," the preacher says, "than to blossom into motherhood."

I was sitting in a plush chair in an echoing room that served as the worship hall for the hip, modern church I chose to attend during college. In an effort to make ancient texts trendy and new, the church was doing a series on modern social topics like abortion, gay marriage, and gender. I was hoping that the church might surprise me, and I was disappointed to discover that the church, despite its bright stage and modern trappings, still thought of women as vessels for birth and considered homosexuals an existential threat.

Submitting to your husband is a godly act, they said, because your husband needs to earn your submission. Things like self-discovery and friendship and education are great, so long as women also understand that our ultimate purpose is reproduction and child-rearing and wifely duties like making dinner or patiently listening to our husbands explain the economy or football or humidifiers. Gay people need our love, they said, to discover the sin that is inherent in their sexual proclivities. Gender is one thing, and sex is another, but either way, the church said, there are only two.

The idea that a life cannot be fulfilling until we are coupled is not a new idea, and it's one that we are culturally fighting against. Rhaina Cohen writes about this extensively in her book *The Other Significant Others*. By de-centering men and our primary relationships, we can find a greater sense of purpose, a supportive community, and more happiness within our primary relationship because our partners aren't expected to fulfill our every need.

Women so often build our lives around men that the way we communicate with each other also centers around men, love, heartache, and relationships. During the year and a half that I was engaged, the way women talked to me was different. Suddenly, I was not a threat to their own relationships. They wanted to see my ring, hear about the proposal, learn about my wedding plans, and share their own relational triumphs and woes. I liked my ring; it had a small diamond with a band that looked like a tree branch. But I didn't like that my fiancé *wasn't* wearing a ring, nor was he expected to. The world didn't know or care that he was engaged, and he was not constantly barraged with questions about the details of our relationship.

I also held the belief that engagements and marriages are final. I grew up believing that with enough hard work and commitment, I could make anything work. That attitude served me well in training, in school, and even later in the workplace. But when it came to relationships, I assumed that if I stuck it out long enough, things would eventually get better. That simply wasn't true. I loved my fiancé very much, but in untangling our union, I learned an important lesson: sometimes, it's healthier to love someone from a distance. Everyone we knew was expecting us to get married. Everyone I met in California knew I was engaged, and I found myself having to explain our anticlimactic dissolution to everyone. Most people did not need or deserve the full backstory, so I would simply say, "it didn't work out," and leave it at that.

A couple weeks after we broke up, I sought the help of a new therapist. Because I had new insurance, I had to see a psychiatrist first, who could match me with the appropriate provider. She asked me a series of questions about myself, my eating disorder, and my relationship. At one point, she gave me a sheet with twenty "yes" or "no" questions and asked me to make my selections.

"Take your time," she told me kindly.

I sat at a small white desk in a large grey office with windows that faced a parking lot and another sleek, grey medical building. I thought about all the time she must sit in this bland office, and in a twisted way, felt bad for this psychiatrist, who had to deal with sadness all day in a building that only amplified ennui and listlessness. Within a matter of minutes, I finished the questionnaire, checking "yes" eighteen times and "no" only twice.

The psychiatrist looked down at the page then up at me, "Do you know what it means to be emotionally abused?" she asked.

I didn't know what to make of this woman, or this office, or my new state of being. "No," I said. I didn't even know what emotional abuse *was*.

"I'm going to have you see Dr. T," the psychiatrist told me. "He works with eating disorder patients, but he can help you with relationships as well. I'm also going to recommend you see a Dietitian. Her name is Amy, and I promise you; you'll love her."

***

When I started seeing Dr. T and Amy the Dietitian, I was past the bad eating disorder stuff: the purging and days of starvation and inevitable binges. My body weight was stable enough that it didn't cause concern, but as anyone with an eating disorder will tell you, the body is only a small part of it. Fixing the real problem requires fixing the brain. I was still standing on the first corner of a Monopoly board, the entire game looming before me.

When I first saw Amy, she asked me if I wanted to weigh myself.

I didn't just say, "No," I said, "*definitely not.*"

Amy was a tall, broad-shouldered woman, a former collegiate swimmer, and a mom. Sometimes you know someone is a mom before you really *know* that they're a mom, and I knew Amy's kids were lucky. She was warm and welcoming, with a big smile, and a quirky but honest way of talking. I saw her every other week, and she slowly but surely dismantled false beliefs I held about food, like that all carbs were bad, or that eating a sweet would make me gain weight.

Amy asked me, every visit, if I wanted to be weighed. She wanted to challenge my fear of the scale and prove to me, with numbers, that my body wouldn't change week to week or meal to meal. Most of all, she wanted to prove to me that weight was nothing to be ashamed of. My body and I had a contentious relationship, and before I entered therapy, I'd weigh myself obsessively, sometimes multiple times per day. I'd get agitated if the scale went up even half a pound and become unreasonably happy if my weight dipped even a bit.

Eventually, I let Amy weigh me but asked that she not tell me what the scale said. I was months into seeing her when I worked up the courage to look down at the scale: 156 pounds.

"How does that feel?" Amy asked. I was expecting to feel shame or disappointment but for some reason, the old familiarity of the scale was replaced by indifference. For the first time in more than a decade, the number meant nothing to me.

"Let me show you something," she said, and with a few clicks of her mouse, my weight fluctuations for nearly a year were before me on a screen.

"What does this all mean?" I asked, squinting, and looking closer. Before Amy could answer, I saw for myself. Each line on the graph represented a pound, and the peaks and valleys were sometimes gentle, increasing a pound or two. Most of the time, the peaks and valleys were nonexistent. For the duration of almost a year, I maintained my weight without even trying. I was shocked. I always assumed I had to fight to lower my weight and keep it low. I believed that I was at war with my body, that without my control tactics, my weight would spiral.

Amy taught me that if I listened to my body and ate intuitively, I would maintain my weight and stay healthy. She also challenged me to eat dessert with her, which I avoided for as long as possible. One day, I walked across the street from my office to the medical building where she worked and saw a cosmic brownie sitting on her desk. My stomach sank and my heart pounded violently in my chest.

"Eat half with me," she suggested.

I was angry at first, resentment coursing through my veins and displaying itself in red splotches across my cheeks. Who was she to think I should eat a brownie, at 10 a.m. no less? My anger was hot and fast and quickly disappeared, like fog when the sun rises. When it did, I was scared. Fear is almost always at the root of my anger, and when it dissipated, I felt foolish. It was a *brownie*, a food I once loved, and I was a fully grown woman. Even still, I couldn't eat it right away and sat staring at the thing as if it were a bomb. At such an early hour, the brownie felt especially indecorous, like laughing at a funeral. We're not supposed to *enjoy* food, I thought, especially not so early in the morning.

Amy took a bite of her half of the brownie, and I gamely took a bite of mine. Tears stung my eyes. I did not like this exercise. I did not like my body. I did not, honestly, like me.

"It's okay," Amy said, putting her brownie down. "It's just food, and food can't hurt you. Remember your weight chart? It hasn't changed for months, and it won't change *if* you decide to eat this brownie."

We took a few deep breaths together before slowly eating our brownies, pinch by chocolate brown pinch. Somewhere in between talking with Amy and taking tiny bites of food, I calmed down, which is not to say I enjoyed the exercise. Guilt and shame soured my stomach, and I thought about going to the gym later to offset these extra calories.

"Did it taste good?" Amy asked.

I considered this. Taste was not something I usually thought about. In fact, I often ate very bland food, like boiled potatoes and canned tuna, exactly because it did *not* taste good. That way, I wouldn't eat too much. But even though I didn't want to eat the brownie, I had to admit that it *did* taste good.

"Yeah," I said. "It wasn't bad."

"Not bad," became my new phrase for everything food related. "Not bad" felt easier than *good*, more accessible, and less scary. If I was ever going to fully shed my eating disorder, I had to shed my fear, and more importantly, I had to shed every voice in my head that instructed me to doubt myself.

Amy and I met for many more months, and I credit the help of a real, certified dietitian for helping me step outside my eating disorder. Therapy helped, but Amy had data and science on her side. She knew how to decipher the ingredients on the back of a cereal box, how much protein was optimal for someone physically active, how food interacts with our bodies, and how much disinformation is out there. I like facts, and when faced with real information about food, my brain struggled to hold onto any belief that was not grounded in fact.

Amy showed me, with detailed graphs and peer-reviewed research papers, how necessary carbohydrates are, especially for athletes. She deconstructed the BMI chart and explained why it's a bad measure of health, especially for muscular bodies. She suggested I get a DEXA scan, which showed my body composition, not just fat and muscle mass but bone density as well. Amy also recommended I read books like *ROAR* by Stacey T Sims, which dove into the nuances of the female body throughout every life cycle. All of this helped relieve my anxiety around food and better understand my body.

I was also learning to listen to my hunger cues, which was eye-opening and uncomfortable. I'd been purposely numbing myself for years and being able to feel both hunger and fullness felt like stepping into a new body. The very last thing Amy and I discussed was another pillar of my diet I'd held onto for far too long: veganism.

VEGAN NO MORE

"Have some orange juice," my father says, plopping a large glass of it down on the Formica-topped table, in front of his bowl of corn flakes that he doused with granulated sugar. I'm visiting home my Junior year of college during the deepest, darkest, dead of winter.

"No thanks," I reply, "I don't really like orange juice."

He raises his eyebrows at me. "Who the hell doesn't like orange juice?" he says, "It's good for you!" He grabs a plate of bacon out of the microwave, "Have some bacon then," he says.

It's piping hot and smells amazing, but I haven't eaten meat in years.

"I can't," I say, with no explanation. It is easier not to over-explain my vegan diet, especially amongst my family. My father used to take my brother deer hunting, and I'd grow jealous of their early morning tromps through the snowy woods. Now, my father goes out for a few days during gun season, but it's my brother who has blossomed into an avid bowhunter, and the bow season is much longer. He routinely kills three, four, even five deer each hunting season, and uses the meat to feed his family. I grew up eating venison too, as well as beef, chicken, pork, you name it. Now, I silently crave meat but deny myself because that's what vegans do. Really, constantly denying oneself is not the trait of a vegan, but of a person with an eating disorder.

My father plops himself onto a scuffed wooden chair and pushes himself up to the table where he proceeds to eat his breakfast. "Well, you'd better eat something," he says, and my mother chimes in, "Yes, shouldn't you eat something, peanut? Before you go running?"

"I'm used to running when I wake up," I answer, but it's a non-answer at best. The weather outside is bitingly cold. My mother eyes me warily, "Stay warm," she says, "if it gets too cold, you can always come back and use the treadmill."

Later, I'll eat black beans and tofu on a plate of iceberg lettuce. I'll eat a few bites before feeding the rest to the dog, who isn't excited about tofu, but eats it anyway. My mother made her infamous homemade pizza for dinner, and since I can't eat cheese or meat, my pizza slice is vegetables and sauce on her chewy, hand rolled crust. It sticks in my throat going down, and I mentally calculate how many carbs are in a single slice of empty pizza. Before I go to bed, I'll open the pantry door to look at all the food I won't allow myself to eat.

***

I didn't go from eating venison and beef to going vegan cold turkey. First, I went to college, where the dorm food was questionable and often made my stomach hurt. I later figured out I was having trouble digesting dairy, like sixty-five percent[5] of the human population. In an effort to solve my stomach woes, I cut out any food with lactose in it and immediately felt legions better.

With dairy, I gave up some of my favorite foods, Greek yogurt, squeaky cheese curds, and soft serve ice cream. Then, I went down a YouTube rabbit hole, finding vegan vloggers who would only eat bananas all day, or who would eat half a watermelon for lunch. Someone gave me a copy of *The China Study*, and I fell for veganism hook, line, and sinker.

I started buying things like nutritional yeast, spirulina powder, chia seeds, tofu, and quinoa. I learned about the pitfalls of factory farming and the dangers meat posed to not only our health, but to the environment. For nearly six years, I held on tight to the idea of myself as a vegan, but I was never entirely convinced that veganism was the best way for me to eat. I just knew it was an easy excuse for why I couldn't eat something in any social situation. As my time in therapy progressed and I distanced myself from my eating disorder, veganism felt less and less wholesome, less fulfilling, and far less healthy.

---

5   "Lactose intolerance," Medline Plus, March 24, 2023, Lactose intolerance: MedlinePlus Genetics

After moving to California, I went to a vegan meet up at a restaurant that served vegan burgers, vegan shakes, and vegan fried chicken. We sat around in circles talking about how healthy we were, how our families "just didn't get it," and dissecting our own unique health routines. One balding, middle-aged man bragged about his fasting routine, how he'd gone up to 48 hours without eating, just drinking water. Another woman in tight, leopard print leggings, talked about a recent family dinner at a restaurant that wasn't very vegan friendly. All they could offer her was a salad, she said, and sides of vegetables. The organizer of the meet-up told me he'd transitioned to veganism after watching *Cowspiracy* on Netflix.

After leaving the restaurant, I realized that I didn't get to know anything about anyone there, other than what they ate, when they ate, or how they arrived at veganism. I also recognized the irony of ingesting look-alike burgers made of soybeans and additives none of us could pronounce. It wasn't a cult, but it was close.

A few weeks later, at my appointment with Amy the dietitian, I told her about a 100k race I had signed up for called Sean O' Brian. The race took place in Malibu the weekend after my birthday, and I thought running 62 miles would be the perfect way to celebrate. I was nervous, I told her, because Sean O'Brian would be my first 100k. Did she have any advice for me about what I should eat?

We chatted about the different types of gels and food commonly offered at long races, and Amy told me to "Eat *often*, and if I were you, I'd eat some real food instead of relying on those gels all day." She was right, as she always was. I ate oranges and bananas and potato chips and chunks of ginger, alongside my standard routine of Cliff Blocks, Gu Roctane gels, and Gatorade. I ran the 100k in 12 hours, 15 minutes and finished in third place for the female category.

In the days after the race, I was overcome by an intense desire for protein. I ate vegan burritos and bowls of quinoa and tofu, but nothing abated my craving. My body was doing its best to recover and demanded protein in a new, more aggressive way. One night, a few days after the race, I dreamed of a thick slab of salmon being roasted over an open fire on a wooden plank. I dreamed about rotisserie chicken, the kind I used to prep and cook when I worked at a grocery store in college, the smell of cooked meat sticking to my skin. I woke up with a dry mouth and an insatiable desire for meat and decided then and there that the jig was up. I stopped by Whole Foods after work, bought an entire rotisserie chicken, and ate it in less than a day.

I felt guilty about eating the chicken, but I also felt *good*.

When I told Amy this, she grinned and said, "That makes *sense*! Your body is trying to rebuild all the muscles you broke down over those 62 miles." She paused to type some notes into my chart before adding kindly, "Eat all the chicken your body needs."

I was expecting her to say, "I told you so, I've *been* telling you so," like my brother would have done when we were kids. I was expecting her to gloat just a bit or express some shock at my sudden dietary change. Instead, she smiled her usual, demure smile and said, "That's great!" just like she would do if I'd told her I'd gotten a pay raise or began putting cream in my coffee again. Everyone in my life had similar reactions when I told them I'd shed my vegan diet. "That's great!" said my friends. "That's great!" said my family. And the world went on merrily spinning, with no regard whatsoever what I put in my mouth or didn't.

WAITING ROOM 2

Dr. T and Amy the Dietitian worked across the street from my office. My workplace was supportive of my need for mental healthcare, so all I had to do was block off an hour of my time on my calendar, no questions asked.

After checking in at the front desk, I'd sit in a waiting room packed with patients. I always saw some of the same people, and I saw them see me, too. None of us was really that different. There was the hyper-obese man who chuckled at the cartoons on the waiting room TV. There was the couple that came and sat, holding hands, waiting for their counseling session. There were the people who came for a group therapy session, who avoided making eye contact with each other until a long woman with dark eyes opened the door and called out, "GROUP!" which prompted them all to stand and saunter through the door behind her. And, the smiling lady at the check-in desk, who gently asked for my insurance card and gave me the same instructions every week: "Fill out this form and leave the iPad with me. You'll go to waiting room 2, down the hall on the right."

Waiting room 2 was *extremely* kid-friendly, with brightly colored floors, one of those roll-around play tables with coiled metal and wooden beads, tiny chairs, and Disney movies playing in the background. My therapist would eventually open the door, call out, "Sarah?" even though I was the only one waiting, and check the television monitor to see which movie was playing, "*The Incredibles* again?" he'd say, shaking his head. I'd walk behind him to his office, where he sat at his desk, a skinny bottle of orange juice next to his computer mouse. I'd sit on the plastic couch adjacent to him, and we'd talk. I'd cry sometimes, or laugh sometimes, or stare blankly out the window as he waited for me to say something.

I was always so tired when I left each session, depleted from all the close examination and questioning. Therapy is hard work, and my therapist routinely called me out for avoiding questions, cracking jokes to ease my tension, or diffusing any of my mental or emotional discomfort with a flippant, "but it doesn't matter." After placing third at Sean O'Brian, I was contacted for an interview for a running website that has since been discontinued.

"What is the accomplishment you're most proud of?" the man who interviewed me asked. He probably meant something about running: a race or a personal record or some pinnacle of athletic success.

By then, I'd ridden many athletic highs and suffered just as many lows. I understood that my time as a healthy athlete was just beginning because by then, I'd learned to feed myself. I was just getting started. So instead, I said, "My proudest accomplishment so far has been recovering from my eating disorder. That's been the hardest thing I've done, by miles."

Recovery was hard because it never really ended. I went back to Waiting Room 2 every other week for nearly two years, and my progress was painfully incremental. Recovery was a constant, daily battle to unlearn my disordered behaviors. It felt gross and uncomfortable, and my body often felt like a foreign entity. Alcoholics celebrate days, months, and years of sobriety. I had no such definitive measure of success. I wanted to get better right away and just be done with it, close the door on my eating disorder and move onto whatever life had in store for me. Instead, I unknowingly entered a years-long process of learning to eat and not hate myself while doing it.

Ultramarathons are hard, anyone will tell you that. But ultras, long as they might seem, don't last forever. Even running for an entire day will eventually fade into a distant memory. When I enter a low point in a race, which always seems to happen, I tell myself that the pain will end. And I repeat my mantra:

you are strong
you are capable
nothing can bring you down

nothing can bring you down
nothing
can
bring
you
down

***

Shortly after I entered therapy, a book arrived on my doorstep, courtesy of Amazon. I purchased it at the recommendation of Amy the Dietitian, who was gently guiding me toward the tall, arched doorways of solid health. What I hadn't initially realized about my eating disorder was that there was a hefty dose of self-loathing sitting at the bottom of it. With Dr. T and Amy, I was unpacking this self-loathing, along with shame, anxiety, disgust, and guilt, negative emotions stacking on top of each other just as quickly as I worked to disassemble them.

Self-love is easy to talk about but difficult to teach. It is easy to assume that once a person's body returns to a normal or healthy size, the eating disorder is gone, but that's not true. My body returned to a healthy size first, and my brain had a lot of catching up to do. The book that landed on my doorstep was called "Neural Rewiring for Eating Disorder Recovery: For real and meaningful mental freedom" by Tabitha Farrar.

The book is short, sweet, and to the point but I'll summarize it to spare you 30 minutes. Our brains create patterns over time, and the pattern of an eating disorder (or any addiction for that matter) can run deep. My eating disorder was formed and re-enforced over many years, so unlearning my behaviors was bound to take a long time and a ton of mental work. Farrar wrote that recovery is hard physically, emotionally, and mentally. The physical part was the easier part because my body was finally nourished. The hard part was mentally grappling with my new body, overcoming the negative emotions I associated with my body and with food, and learning new ways to exist that didn't include my eating disorder. As I read the book, I felt disheartened by how far I still had to go and reassured by the fact that my long recovery timeline was normal. Immediate changes are far less likely to stick than changes made over a long period of time. If I could just move a few grains of sand every day, I would eventually be standing at the beach.

"How did you like the book?" Amy the Dietitian asked me the following week.

"It was fine," I answered carefully, "but how exactly am I supposed to create new pathways in my brain? It all seems so vague and so," I threw my hands up in defeat, "*slow.*"

"It might be helpful to dissociate your recovery with any specific timeline," she said. "This will be a process. You can't rush it. But you *can* celebrate your victories. Even the very small ones." She was fiddling with a plastic ice cream cone, one of her many props to talk to clients about their fear foods.

One day, we sorted each food toy into categories: good and bad. The fruits and vegetables went in the good pile. Sweets of any kind went in the bad. Some things, like eggs or meat or yogurt, went in a separate, third pile that I didn't know how to categorize. After I sorted my fear foods, Amy looked at them for a moment before mixing them all back together.

How *dare* she, I thought, furrowing my brow.

"Now, imagine all these foods without a label. Not good. Not bad. Just, food. And pick out whichever food you'd like to have right now, in this moment."

Because it was plastic food, I chose the ice cream cone. It was white with colorful sprinkles, and I thought about how long it had been since I'd eaten real ice cream or enjoyed it. Even though it was only 10 a.m., and I knew the food wasn't real, I hated that I'd chosen the ice cream cone.

"Good," Amy said, and that was that.

INTUITIVE EATING

Amy the Dietitian taught me many things, but perhaps the most valuable was intuitive eating. Intuitive eating, she told me, is not just eating whatever you want whenever you want. Intuitive eating is about listening to what your body needs. If your body needs a burger, eat the burger. If you're full halfway through the burger, stop eating the burger. If your body wants leafy greens, give it leafy greens. If your body is dehydrated, drink some water, and maybe add some electrolytes. Take time to pay attention to what you eat. Take time to feel your hunger and your fullness. Intuitive eating has been scrutinized and bastardized, but it is not complicated. Eat well, listen to your body, and *take your time*.

It was weird to tune into my body because I was so used to tuning *out*. You can't hear a song if the volume is on zero. Suddenly, I was asked to notice not only the song, but the tempo, rhythm, and lyrics.

I had many tricks to keep my eating disorder on track. I learned to disconnect from my hunger pains and that caffeine could calm them, for a while. I learned to eat voluminous foods that offered few calories: iceberg lettuce, raw carrots, watermelon. I learned to stay so busy that I didn't have time to think about food. And worst of all, I learned exactly how to make myself throw up quickly, the exact spot I could press on the back of my tongue to ignite my gag reflex. I learned that I could make myself feel sick if I drank enough water, so I'd momentarily feel uninclined to eat. I learned that I would fall asleep eventually if I ignored my nightly hunger pains. And if I couldn't sleep, a teaspoon of peanut butter or a melatonin tablet usually helped.

I kept measuring spoons handy, so I knew exactly how much oatmeal I boiled, or exactly how much cereal I poured, or exactly how much brown rice I mixed with my broccoli and tofu. Before I had an eating disorder, I assumed that someone with Anorexia never ate at all, but that isn't true. Most of us eat, at least sometimes. We have to. It can be hard for Anorexics to admit they have a problem because the result of starving is often a culturally-condoned thinness. To the world, I looked like I was winning.

We need food just as badly as we need air and water and sleep and love. I had safe foods like apples, carrots, and tofu. I also avoided many foods, like bread, sweets, anything full of carbs, meat, or anything I perceived to be fatty, oily, or fried. I ate the same "safe" foods every day, and if something or someone got in the way of my morning carafe of coffee, I became extremely agitated. I was starving myself, but I needed to starve on my own terms; that's how my eating disorder manifested. Some people eat very little, or only eat one food, or binge. Eating disorders aren't all the same, and even though I suffered from one, I didn't understand the many ways any mental disorder can manifest.

I still don't, because it's difficult for humans to experience nuance. It's easier, and often correct, to categorize people, places, and realities so we can understand the world to some degree. But categories are limiting, and beliefs can serve as blinders. I categorized myself as healthy, even though I was killing myself. I never believed I would be the kind of person to fall into a mental illness because I thought of myself as strong and thought of mental illnesses as weak. This was a belief I'd either found or been given, picked up like a dollar bill on a sidewalk or spoon fed like applesauce. Easy to swallow, and sweet going down.

I didn't understand what I was experiencing because my paradigm didn't make room for nuance. The world I was born into was black and white, cut and dry. Things were either good or bad. People were either good or bad. Food was either good or bad. *Life* was either good or bad.

So, when Amy started teaching me to eat intuitively, I was *very* uncomfortable. Discomfort was only on the surface of it though. Sometimes, it felt so bad and so dangerous to be in my body that I thought it might just be easier to die. I had tuned my body out for so long that I didn't understand, in a real, tangible sense, what my body needed.

When I started running ultramarathons, I was no longer clinically underweight. I'd regained some muscle mass, so taking on a longer distance wasn't unhealthy, necessarily. What I struggled with the most was eating and drinking *while* running. I read books and articles about the science of nutrition, how many carbs to ingest every hour, how much water, and what types of electrolytes. I spoke with other runners, trying to glean some idea of what I should do, how much I should eat, and how often. But my brain was still stuck in my eating disorder, and I continuously bonked while training, my muscles depleted of glycogen, my body functionally shutting down. I'd go out for a 20-mile trail run with one gel and 16 ounces of water. I thought that sports gels were bad because they were packed with sugar, and started eating dates or Lara bars, which only upset my stomach. After running, I wouldn't feel hungry all day and skipped important recovery meals, nausea and exhaustion getting in the way of me being able to rest or perform.

Amy did her best to help me. "You need fuel for these long adventures!" she'd exclaim. "Your body is burning so much fuel!" She directed me to sports nutrition resources, and I halfheartedly pursued them, believing that I knew better.

Finally, I hit a minor breaking point: a trail marathon up in Big Bear, CA. Big Bear sits 6,700 feet above sea level, and I didn't realize it at the time, but running at elevation presents more complex challenges than running at sea level, like quicker dehydration, more intense exposure to sun, and a greater chance of experiencing nausea. The marathon took me just over five hours to complete, and I bonked extremely hard. It was a hot day, and I wore a hydration vest that held a two-liter bladder of water. I carried one Lara bar and a plastic baggy holding three dates. I was wearing a long sleeve sun shirt to shield my skin from the glaring sun. By all measures, I *looked* like I knew what I was doing, but I was as green as a crocus leaf, and inexperienced as a newborn.

I wasn't drinking enough water (my first mistake) and when I ate my Lara bar, over halfway into the race, my stomach immediately turned (mistake number two). After pooping behind a tree,

I jogged a few miles to the next aid station, where I thirstily drank a tiny paper cup of coke, then another, and another.

After finishing the race, I hugged my friend Steve who was there manning a vendor booth. "You did great!" he said. "I feel awful," I answered.

He just laughed and offered me his chair. Feeling awful is a trail running rite of passage, and he delighted in my misery, pounding my back while pumping his fist.

I gratefully took the chair he offered and immediately started shaking: a classic sign of dehydration. I hadn't eaten enough, and Lara Bars were not the right fuel for me. They contained too much fiber, and I had run myself sick. Instead of enjoying my race, I began wondering why I continuously put myself through such extreme discomfort. I also wondered about the other runners I saw crossing the finish line, in a wide meadowed area surrounded by large, ponderosa pines. How did they all look *okay*, albeit tired? Why wasn't anyone else sitting shivering in a camping chair? Why did they all look so *happy*?

I walked to my car and sat with the heat blasting until I felt a bit better. The drive home was two hours, the first hour down a winding mountain road. I stopped at a gas station in town and bought two bottles of Gatorade. By the time I got home, it was all I could do to shower and fall into bed. My entire body felt like I'd turned it inside out and scratched each of my muscles with a bristle brush.

The next week, Amy told me, "I'm concerned about you doing these long races without eating. It's not healthy for you."

I knew she was right, and I also knew exactly what I was doing wrong. I needed to eat, and I needed to figure out what my body could handle eating. Nutrition isn't rocket science, but here I was, making it seem like the most difficult task in the world.

To figure out what would help me feel better on race day, I started carrying water with me when I trained. On runs that were longer than an hour, I'd also eat Cliff blocks, at least 2 every 30 minutes. I'd bring peanut butter and honey sandwiches with me during long runs and found that I finished runs feeling good instead of feeling turned inside out. The difference between feeling strong and feeling terrible was as simple as eating, and the correlation between food and performance crystallized. My entrance into the world of ultramarathons necessarily collided with my ability to finally, *finally* eat enough.

WHAT DOESN'T MAKE YOU STRONGER

Amelia Boone, a spartan and ultra endurance athlete, has this famous quote, "I'm not the strongest. I'm not the fastest. But I'm really good at suffering." She later redacted this statement, stating that "enduring" is a more fitting word than "suffering." Before she made this clarification, I never thought about the difference. To endure is to suffer, but with patience. To endure is to know that you will, at some point, exit the suffering.

I didn't realize it until I was hip-deep in hurt, but I was good at suffering, too. Running hard brought me an immediate physical sensation of discomfort and sometimes, pain. The more I leaned into that pain the less I could bear to think about anything else. Running became a crutch that taught me to endure the difficult parts of life, and life has taught me that there will always, always be difficulty.

I asked Dr. T one day if pain is a good motivator. "It's the only thing that works for me," I said, "Like, I just don't really know any other way to motivate myself to succeed."

He thought for a moment and answered, "I'm not an athlete like you so I can't say for sure, but it seems like an exhausting incentive, like always having a chip on your shoulder. At some point, internal motivation needs to be stronger than the external stuff because the external stuff will stop working."

"How do you *know* it will stop working?" I asked, pushing him for details. I needed to know that giving up my eating disorder wouldn't hurt my ability to run hard or fast. I needed to know that I would still be able to push myself if I wasn't choosing to hurt myself.

He looked at me over his round glasses. "You're here, aren't you?" he said. "I think that's enough. You seem like you want to resolve your distress but you're afraid that without it, you won't be *you* anymore. Is that right?"

I would normally answer a question like this with a pout, or by averting my eyes. I hated when Dr. T said something true. "That's right," I said, jutting my chin out stubbornly.

Then he said something that has stuck with me ever since, something I wrote on a sticky note and stuck to my desk so I'd have to see it every day, read it every day, and eventually believe it to be true.

"You can be a badass without constantly suffering," he said, "hurting all the time doesn't necessarily make you stronger."

RETURNING

After Chad and I moved to Southern California, we met a group of trail runners who met once a week at a local state park. These were not your run-of-the-mill casual 5k'ers either. Every week, they'd run between five and twelve miles, depending on daylight and overall group sentiment. There was a group that ran long and a group that ran short, and the people I met at the park every Wednesday were warm and welcoming and entirely unbothered with pace or mile splits. After the run, they would hang around and drink beer, cracking jokes and causing a ruckus. The group drew people of all ages, and if I hadn't met them, running might have become a distant memory, one I'd look back fondly on when I was flipping through old photos or feeling nostalgic.

By the time I arrived in California, I'd already decided to stop running. "It just doesn't bring me any joy anymore," I told one of my therapists in Chicago, "it feels like a chore." And it did. Every time I bundled up to head out the door for a run in Chicago's deep winter freeze, I hated every moment and dreaded every step. The monotony of running made my eyes glaze over and any of the meditative pleasure I'd found in running earlier in my life had dried up into a hard, crusty ball of disdain.

"You don't ever have to run again," my therapist told me, "But you might also find happiness in it someday, and I encourage you to remain open to that."

I listened without believing what she said, and by the time Chad and I landed in Southern California, I'd given away bags of running clothes and shoes that I no longer used, figuring I'd no longer need them. We ended up in the Orange County suburb of Aliso Viejo, and our apartment was only a mile away from a lush canyon cut through with dozens of trails. The top of the trail overlooked a park called "Top of the World," where you could see Laguna Beach, the never-ending Pacific, and on clear days, Catalina Island in the distance. There were mountains a half hour drive away and even taller mountains just a few dozen miles further. California is home to an endlessly diverse landscape that's accessible nearly year-round. Like kids in a candy shop, we began exploring the trails and mountains, and I felt my old love for running rise from the ashes, a bit rusted and unfamiliar, like a childhood friend that somehow grew into adulthood without my noticing.

I started waking up early to run on the trails before work, relishing the quiet mornings I spent alone with my thoughts as I watched the sunrise. I continued to run as much as I wanted, whenever I wanted, until I decided to train for ultramarathons. But then, about a year after I stood on the podium at Kodiak holding the carved wooden bear, the COVID-19 pandemic put a screeching halt to day-to-day life.

At the time, I was working in fundraising for the American Red Cross, and my office job suddenly went fully remote. I had dozens of unused vacation days saved and began to feel stifled by the stay-at-home order. I *understood* that staying at home could prevent the spread of Covid, but I also *needed* to move, to be outside in nature and not cooped up in my bedroom in an apartment I shared. I began exercising excessively, an old habit brought back on by boredom and stress. In addition to running, I bought an indoor bike and began cycling while binging Netflix. I started drinking wine every night out of boredom and going for long walks on the trail system that backed the apartment complex.

During the pandemic, I envied my parents for their large yard and lush gardens, their 120 acres of forests and fields. I envied the swamp, the creek, the wild apricots that grew along the fence line and the clean, unobstructed air. It would be easy to isolate at home, I thought. I even briefly considered moving back to Wisconsin to grab a chunk of land for myself. But the mountains were calling, and I was not done making my acquaintance.

***

During the pandemic, the days melted together in dystopian greyscale. In an effort to wake myself out of the COVID slumber, I took a random Thursday off work to do a double summit up a nearby mountain. Mount San Antonio, or Mount Baldy, sits just over 10,000 feet. At the time, I had never double summited Mount Baldy before, but I climbed it often so I could easily measure my progress. Mount Baldy is a popular mountain, its proximity to Los Angeles making it an easy escape for millions of people who may or may not be adequately prepared. That Thursday, the parking lot was empty, and I was giddy at the thought of having the mountain to myself.

I started at Manker Flat, running up a fire road, past the ski lodge, up the infamous Devil's Backbone and reached the summit breathless. I saw a few hikers along the way, and waved as I ran past, chirping a perky, "Good morning!" The first summit was feeling effortless. *I can do anything,* I thought. I trotted down the mountain slowly in an effort to save my quads for the return trip up. Back in the parking lot, I made a pit stop at my car to refill my pack with water and snacks. My pack held two liters of water, but the day was growing hot, and two liters would turn out to be not enough. By the time I reached the summit a second time, I was out of water and my throat was tacky. As I stood on the summit calculating how long it would take me to run back to my car, a hiker stopped in his tracks and asked, "Weren't you just running down?"

"I was," I answered, giving him a nod.

"Well, what are you training for?" he asked.

I paused because there was nothing I *was* training for. Every race I'd signed up for that year was canceled, so I just shrugged and said, "Not a thing."

As I started descending the mountain, I remembered something my friend Ben had told me, that you're okay for about two hours without water, but beyond that, you can start to really have problems. Each summit and return would take roughly three hours, and normally, there is a ski lodge halfway down the mountain where runners and hikers can refill their water. However, due to COVID, the lodge was closed. I circled the building a few times like a rabid animal, desperately searching for a hose or outdoor spigot. There was nothing. I continued down the mountain, finding a small stream a while later and sipping from that. It was unfiltered mountain water, which is risky on a good day, but I didn't care. I arrived back at my car sunburned, exhausted, thirsty, and famished, but undeniably stoked. The aching sensation in my legs would fade, but in the meantime, I absolutely glowed.

A couple weeks later, my friend Alex found a race near Beaver, Utah that was green-lighted despite COVID-19. There was a half marathon, marathon, 70K, and 100K distance. *You in?* he asked.

Absolutely. I signed up for the 100k, before finding out that he had signed up for the 70K.

Wait, why didn't you sign up for the 100? I texted him, *don't tell me you're getting soft.*

He typed back, *did you check the elevation profile?*

Well no, I hadn't. The race is called Tushars, and it starts at 10,000 feet. There are about 17,000 feet of climbing over 62 miles, and runners never dip below 8,000 feet. At the time, I was living three miles from the ocean, and cringed thinking about how my sea-level lungs would struggle in the thin air. But now my pride was on the line.

It'll be fine, I told Alex. And it was, sort of.

The race started early, with waves of runners standing six feet apart. I was the only one in my wave who wasn't carrying poles, because I didn't have any and didn't think I'd need them. One of the required items was a rain jacket, which I tied to the outside of my pack because it wouldn't fit inside. As the race started, I intentionally went slow, knowing I would struggle with the elevation. Twenty miles in, I felt myself struggling to breathe, but that wasn't my biggest problem. My stomach had turned from the altitude, leaving me gagging and throwing up on the side of the mountain, bitter bile sticking to the back of my tongue and reminding me of the dozens of times I'd kneeled over a toilet bowl with my fingers down my throat, feeling the exact same way.

My throat constricted with a mixture of grief and frustration. Would I ever be able to think about my past with utter indifference? I longed to recall bouts of starving and binging and purging with the same apathy I normally reserved for mandatory workplace sexual harassment trainings or church services or medical claims. This time, I was not sick because I wanted to be though, I was sick because of altitude, and there was nothing I could do about it.

At the 20-mile aid station, I saw my friend Dave, who was there to pace my other friend, Jesse. "How are you feeling?" he said, beaming. Dave is one of the nicest humans on the planet, always willing to pace or crew other runners, always supportive, and always smiling. Today, his smile felt only a little infuriating.

"I keep throwing up," I answered. "I feel awful." Dave knew not to give me an out or too much sympathy. He went into problem-solving mode, mixing some liquid nutrition called Tailwind into one of my bottles and instructing me to drink it.

"This will give you easy calories," he said. "Drink all of this and I'll refill your bottle so you can take some with you. I hear there's a big climb ahead."

We had to run 10 miles out and another 10 miles back to this same aid station. I told myself I could muscle it out and at the very least make it back here. Then, I might allow myself to drop out of the race. I started playing little games with myself, seeing how long I could wait to check my watch, counting my steps until I lost track, seeing if I could remember all the lyrics to a Colter Walls song, "Sleeping on the Blacktop," which incidentally, sounded like a nice, relaxing, and totally normal activity in the moment.

Sometimes, I can't remember an entire song and my brain will replay the same lyric repeatedly, *coyotes chewing on a cigarette pack o' young boys going howlin' at the moon.* Sometimes I think of a poem I've written, or just lines of a poem, like, "when you learn how to eat again, eat / tattoo a lotus on your bicep to celebrate life / when someone asks what it means say / 'I almost died, but I didn't' / just to see their surprise."

Sometimes I think about my past or my future, but most of the time I'm stuck in the moment. How long has it been since I've eaten? How much water have I had? Is my body painful in a bad way or is it just the expected aching? Is my stomach upset? Are my limbs frying to a crisp? As I slowly made my way through the out and back, I went from feeling terrible to feeling kind of okay, then back to terrible again. When I got back to the same aid station hours later, I felt my mental fortitude wane. "I think I need to drop," I told a woman at the aid station.

She looked at me for a long second before answering, "You *can* finish this race. You just don't *think* you can."

She was right, and I knew it and hated that I knew it. I had stopped vomiting by then, and food was going down easier. I was tired and beaten up, but I wasn't injured. There was no reason for me to stop, aside from the fact that I really wanted to. I sat for a few minutes, eating slices of candied ginger and salty potato chips. Some of the aid station workers were trying to lift my spirits, cracking jokes, and having their own fun. But I wasn't ready for jokes, I was uncomfortable and trying to grapple with the prospect of even more discomfort. Probably another eight hours of it.

One man asked me if I wanted to ride back to the finish line. I was relieved and ashamed as I answered, "Yes." I immediately felt regret lurch in my chest and quickly changed my mind. "Nevermind!" I told him, and started trotting down the mountain, the aid station volunteers cheering behind me. I would have to climb back up this mountain in the dark, my feeble headlamp shining dimly in the deep forest. I presumed that spending an entire day mostly alone in the mountains would be an open invitation for all my inner demons to rise to the surface, but the longer I spent with myself, the more my demons began to seem less like monsters and more like misunderstood children.

As I started the largest climb of the race, a 4,000-foot ascent up the backside of the mountain, I briefly cursed at myself for not bringing poles. My legs were heavy, and I put my hands on my knees, pushing on my own body to gain leverage. Halfway up the mountain, I felt wetness between my legs and realized I'd started my period. I didn't have a tampon with me, so I thanked my lucky stars that I'd chosen black shorts that morning. As I climbed and climbed and climbed, I thought about the six years I'd spent living without a period and how long it took to get my period back. Now that it had returned, I clung to its subtleties, the way my energy dipped and surged throughout the month, the way my skin broke out the week before I bled, the way I socialized one week before becoming a recluse the next. I felt more feminine now, more like a woman and less like an adolescent girl. I laughed out loud as I bled through my shorts, pulling my phone out to log the start of my cycle in my period tracking app. Anything can happen on the side of a mountain.

The last third of my race was tough, but by then, I'd surpassed the worst mental hurdles and clicked off each remaining mile. Thirteen, twelve, eleven, ten. The last aid station was eight miles from the finish line. A man sat in the back of a tent on a cot, sipping vegetable soup and trying to warm up.

"Are you okay?" I asked him, taking a cup of soup myself.

"I'm just trying to warm up before I get back out there," he answered, giving me the smallest smile.

I could see myself in his face, so I told him what the volunteers had told me earlier, "You *can* finish this race." I offered him my emergency blanket and headed back into the night.

As I ran and hiked the last eight miles, I made a game of finding the next course marker, orange glowing ribbons shining in the deep purple dark. When I crossed the finish line, shortly after 2:00 a.m., I grinned, tears stinging the corners of my eyes. I gave Alex a hug, and greeted my friend Laura, who waited up into the early morning hours to see me cross the finish line.

"I can't believe it," I cried as I threw my arms around Alex. And even though I'd been there the whole time, it still struck me as unbelievable. Only a few years ago, I'd been clinically malnourished and gave up on the thought of ever running a race again. And yet, there I was, with people who loved me, doing the exact thing I'd never, until then, been strong enough to endure.

ANXIOUS-AVOIDANT ATTACHMENT

"So he ghosts me, right?," I tell my therapist, "After eight months, this man has the nerve to ghost me." I pull both of my legs to my chest before letting them fall back to the floor with a heavy thud. "And then! Two weeks go by and he calls me professing his love. That's so fucked *up*."

"Have you heard about attachment styles?" Dr. T asks, setting down his skinny plastic bottle of orange juice.

"Sort of," I answered. "But I always thought they were kind of bullshit. Like astrology."

He chuckles, which makes me happy. Humor is an easy buffer, a handy tool I've used for a long time to heighten my likability while maintaining emotional distance. My self-awareness of this has done little to change my behavior, and I figure it's better to be a little fucked up and likable rather than to be simply fucked up.

"Attachment theory began in the 1950's," Dr. T tells me, "And it's been validated countless times, unlike astrology. Knowing your attachment style can't fix your relationship woes, but it may help you become aware of your behaviors, and eventually, change them."

He has a tiny, two-drawer filing cabinet on wheels from which he occasionally extracts informational handouts. The last one he gave me had the face of a small boy crying splayed across the page along with the unfortunate title, "Coping with Emotional Distress." I kept it in the bottom of my backpack for a week before reading its crumpled pages on the toilet one morning.

This time, he offers me a small, folded pamphlet with "Attachment Styles" typed neatly across the page. "Take this home and fill it out," he tells me. "We'll talk about your results next week."

Later that same evening, I sat in bed with my cat and completed the assessment. When I finished, I learned I'm something called "anxious avoidant," which is basically two bad attachment styles smashed into one. My results read, verbatim, "A person with anxious-avoidant attachment lives in an ambivalent state, in which they are afraid of being both too close or too distant from others. The person they want to go to for safety is the same person they are frightened to be close to. As a result, they have no organized strategy for getting their needs met by others."

That last line hit a soft spot in my stomach. Months ago, when I was using Bumble to get back in the dating scene, one of the prompts I answered was, "Who holds you accountable?" and my not-so-cryptic answer was, "Myself." A verifiable anxious-avoidant, scouring the dark world of online dating for a boring date and a tall glass of chardonnay.

When I took my results to Dr. T at our next appointment, he was not shocked, to say the least. I ignored his knowing look and asked what I thought would be an easy question to answer, "So, where do these attachment styles come from exactly?"

"They are, first and foremost, formed in infancy and can be taught or un-taught throughout childhood or your teenage years." What he meant is that I could fully and completely blame my parents (not really). "Anxious-avoidant attachment styles are a doozy," he said.

And here's why: anxious attachment styles are formed in childhood by infants who receive love and care *unpredictably*. These people often have a positive view of others, but a negative view of themselves. They depend heavily on others for their own self-esteem. In contrast, avoidant attachment styles are developed by infants who only have some of their needs met. For instance, they may be fed enough but not held enough. Avoidant types have a positive view of themselves and a negative view of others. They are astutely independent and don't rely on others for emotional support.

I'm at a bit of a loss here. Anxiousness and avoidance seem diametrically opposed. I look up at the soft tiled ceiling, wondering if this man is actually helping me.

Dr. T assures me that, "Attachment styles can change. It's fully possible to develop a healthy, secure style."

"*How*?" I ask, with so much blunt force that he laughs out loud. He smiles in a way that is entirely unbothered, which irks me for some reason. I was starting to catch on, though. I'm at once a frustrated driver and the pedestrian who decides to stop in the middle of the street to send a text. I'm both the lazy employee and the exasperated manager. I am the child who craved attention and the child who wriggled away from a comforting embrace.

I feel a memory resurface from the cold, dusty recesses of my unconscious. Growing up, I was obsessed with crafting, likely a side effect of having little else to do. I painted rocks, completed paint-by-numbers, learned to sew, learned to weave, learned to bead, and knit and watercolor and macramé. One Christmas, my mother gave me tea towels with quaint birds outlined in the corners and fabric paint to color them in. I set about my task with concentration, spreading my project across many days to make the craft "last" before I was forced to find a new one.

One day after school, I arrived home to an empty house and began completing one of the bird tea towels. But almost immediately, I ruined the whole thing by squeezing a huge, ugly glob of green paint over a large portion of the quaint bird, not on purpose. Many kids wouldn't have cared, and many more would have just started over with a new towel. But 10-year-old-me was distraught. I remember crying on the staircase until my mother came home and comforted me, assuring me that the towel didn't matter and that everything would be okay.

I shared this memory with my therapist, who simply said, "It sounds like you wanted to paint the towel well, and the failure to do so was devastating. Maybe," and here he leaned closer to me, "you got the message somewhere along the way that doing things well would earn you the love you craved but couldn't access elsewhere. Or maybe you were, or *are*, unable to let yourself access it elsewhere." As he said this, with a small smile on his calm face, I desperately wanted to punch him. I wanted the words he said to not be true so badly that I knew they *must* be true. That's the difficult part about therapy; it isn't a place to go and vent frustration, though that is part of it. It's a place where we decode the parts of us that are broken, greet them with love, and figure out how to reshape ourselves in a way that isn't quite as pointed and abrasive. I knew he was right. The desire to do well, to achieve things and be recognized for achievement, turns out to be one of the most telling signs of anxious-avoidant attachment.

I'm not exactly sure how to go about fixing this, but as Dr. T assures me, knowing my style and wanting to change it is a critical first step. He tells me I will need to practice recognizing my anxious-avoidant behaviors, like getting attached to a romantic partner, then pushing them away when the relationship feels too vulnerable, then desperately trying to re-establish the connection I just pushed away. One morning, I told Dr. T. about a guy I met through Instagram, "I don't like when he doesn't communicate," I say. "But then, if he communicates too much, I feel icky, and I start hating him."

"It sounds like you maybe just don't like this guy that much," Dr. T. posits. "Have you thought about that? If you actually like him?"

I pause to ponder, because I don't know if I actually like him or not. "I like that he likes me, I guess," I answer. "And I like when he comes back."

Dr. T. leans back in his chair, his round belly threatening to pop out of his tucked in polo shirt. "Perfect," he says. "We're going to start there. I want you to first determine if you like this guy as a person. If you do, we'll work on how to improve your communication. If you don't, we'll work on how to set boundaries so that you don't feel like you need to engage with people you don't like."

A few weeks later, I ended things with the man from Instagram. "It felt terrible," I told Dr. T. "I felt so mean. He *cried*. And now I feel like I miss him."

"You don't miss him," Dr. T. tells me. "You're just missing the ups and downs you created for yourself. You're missing the chaos. But this won't happen next time, because next time, you won't let it get this far."

I groan out loud at the very thought of "next time." I didn't have the heart to try to date anyone anymore, it felt like too much time and too much mental energy. I'm tired to the bone, and it's only 11 a.m. But, as a kitschy poster over Dr. T's gray, plastic couch reads, "Nothing in this life is permanent."

SAD, BEAUTIFUL WOMEN

"Have you been avoiding me?" Dr. T asks as he fetches me from Waiting Room 2. We walk down a long, beige hallway to his sparsely furnished office. As I plop onto a cheap foam couch adjacent to his desk, I wonder how many other people have sat on this exact cushion. The thought strikes me as sad. Dr. T is nearing retirement (so he says), and the frequency with which he mentions this is truly alarming. He always wears all-black converse that zip up the side; I find this odd at his age, but of course I say nothing.

"Maybe," I respond, although the real answer is *yes*. Definitely. Of course, I've been avoiding him, skipping my last two scheduled sessions because I've felt increasingly terrible, and the last thing I want to do when I feel terrible is talk to someone about it.

He quirks an eyebrow at me, "And why is that?"

Dr. T specializes in eating disorders, and I see him because I've had an eating disorder for a very long time. "A very long time" is a vague way of saying nearly half my life. I don't know why I started "having" an eating disorder, but I'm willing to bet it's a lot like coming down with skin cancer, or diabetes. Nobody can really point to the exact moment in time their bodies begin metastasizing, just like I cannot point to the exact moment in time I decided to starve myself. In the grand scheme of things, the inception doesn't really matter.

Because Dr. T specializes in eating disorders, I don't feel like I should talk to him about anything else, even though my eating disorder is the last thing that has recently burdened my mind.

"Lately, I haven't felt like eating," I tell him. "Actually, I don't feel like doing *anything*." This last part is undeniable; I can't concentrate on work; I can't concentrate on reading. I don't even feel like watching TV and find the effort of scrolling through the endless options cruelly daunting. Despite constant exhaustion, I can't fall asleep. I tell him all of this, pinching the soft spot between my left thumb and pointer finger with my right thumb and pointer finger. Someone once told me that this spot is a pressure point, and I should press on it hard when I have a headache. I never have headaches, but it feels good to press it just the same.

Therapy is objectively weird. It is weird to sit in a tiny, dimly lit room and divulge my grossest thoughts to a near stranger. It's very uncomfortable, and I normally wouldn't admit to my discomfort, but Dr. T is staring at my hands, so I say, "This is really uncomfortable."

He looks at me calmly, shaking his head *yes*, and I can't shake the feeling that he's a lot like my cat; content and happy in the ray of sunlight beaming through his office window.

"It sounds like you're experiencing an episode of minor depression," he says.

"But why?"

"Why not?"

It is easy to believe that everything happens for a reason. I like to imagine that every cause has a cut and dry effect, and that the aftershocks of one event gently recede into the ether instead of igniting another quake. Life is more chaos than order and even though I know this, I can't help but feel like it would be nice if we could just circle back to the chaos next week, when I'm more rested and less listless and have some semblance of hope again.

I've felt down before, yes, but never uninspired to get out of bed. Never this relentless hopelessness that seems unfounded to outsiders, and even to myself. I have an objectively good life, with a good, fulfilling job, good people who care about me, a safe home in a beautiful city, a sweet cat and the ability to chase any of my impractical dreams.

Sometimes, there is no single reason for feeling down or blue or even depressed. Often, there is no simple, straightforward way to feel better, either.

Dr. T is able, though, to drill down on one specific point: my lack of sleep.

"Sleep is incredibly important," he tells me. I know this. He knows this. Everyone who has an eighth of a brain knows that sleep is important. I make a mental note to later make a toast to my exorbitantly low co-pay in celebration of not paying for such pedestrian advice.

"When depressed people can't sleep, their depressive symptoms worsen," he says. "Try listening to a podcast or audio book that's marginally compelling. Something interesting enough to capture your attention, but uninteresting enough that you're also a bit bored."

I was not enthused with this advice, but I had literally nothing to lose.

That night, after getting home late from a work event, drinking half a glass of chardonnay and eating a roasted yam, I found myself curled up in bed with Chub Chub, unable to sleep. My mind went from worrying about work, to finances, to Thanksgiving, to the weekend, to my car's dented bumper, to drowning, to my blog, to my shopping list (can't forget laundry detergent), to a poem I recently wrote.

After an hour of manic thinking and a bit of CBD that had no effect on my drowsiness, I opened Audible and downloaded Henry David Thoreau's, *Civil Disobedience and Other Essays*, in search of the following quote:

> *The mass of men lead lives of quiet desperation. What is called resignation is confirmed desperation. From the desperate city you go into the desperate country and have to console yourself with the bravery of minks and muskrats. A stereotyped but unconscious despair is concealed even under what are called the games and amusements of mankind. There is no play in them, for this comes after work. But it is a characteristic of wisdom not to do desperate things.*

If you ever have trouble sleeping, I highly recommend listening to an 1849 collection of essays on resisting civil government. You will find it impossible to stay awake. I promise.

***

I was with Chad for over five years, so when I started dating again, I didn't know what the hell I was doing. I trusted men (and everyone, for that matter) blindly. I treated men on dating apps as if they were human, and they treated me as if I were red meat. I didn't know how to tell if a man was lying to me, I didn't have a clue what to put on a dating profile, and I didn't know that I should say, "I'll buy my own drink, thank you though," to the random men who offered me endless glasses of Jack and Coke.

After I downloaded Bumble, then deleted it in favor of Hinge, I noticed a pattern called *men will say anything if they think it'll get them laid*. Dozens of men told me how stunningly gorgeous I was, which I knew right off the bat was shady because although I have a solid facial structure, I'm no runway model. Sometimes, I pretended to be stupid just to play with them or tell them awful jokes to see how they'd respond. Sometimes I'd make up elaborate back stories that involved a family vineyard in the south of France, or a degree in archaeology, or an intense interest in Sheba Inus. Most of the men I met were nice enough, but they all tended to blend together in a hazy soup of neutral toned collared shirts and talk of cryptocurrency.

When I expressed frustration about online dating to Dr. T, he told me, "You have what I call the 'curse of attractiveness.' Many women, especially women in the [eating disorder] program, have this. It's an interesting phenomenon."

What the fuck, I thought. *Did my therapist just hit on me??*

He wasn't hitting on me (thank God) and explained that pretty women are often valued only for their looks, so we grow up thinking that our looks are all that matter. Even though (duh), that's not true, it's everywhere we look. I was only 27 at the time, but already the fear of aging was tugging at my subconscious. Aging makes men steamier and women sadder, apparently.

Dr. T and I talked about how and why beautiful women are sad. For one, because we learned, from a very young age, that how we look is more important than how we think, what we know, or what we can do. This is a curse because we don't *want* to be valued for how we look; looks fade, always. This is a curse because people assume that attractive people *must* be happy. What more could a beautiful girl ask for? We are sad, sometimes, because we are *expected* to be happy. We are expected to know that we're beautiful and for that to be enough.

Some of the most successful, powerful women to ever live are continually judged by how they look. We talk about their hair, their outfits, and their skincare routines, instead of focusing on their talents or skills, or on the work they are doing.

A story in the April 2012 issue of *Elle* magazine quoted Hilary Clinton's aides bemoaning her habit of pulling her hair back in a casual ponytail with a scrunchie. "Her hair, a perennial topic, and makeup, or lack thereof, have been in the news since the Drudge Report posted a photo of the Secretary of State wearing glasses and no cosmetics other than lipstick during a trip to India."

Asked about the attention in an interview on CNN, Clinton said she is beyond worrying about anyone's reaction to her appearance. "If I want to wear my glasses, I'm wearing my glasses. If I want to wear my hair back, I'm pulling my hair back. You know at some point it's just not something that deserves a lot of time and attention." Her response led to a flurry of media from newspapers, morning news shows, and blogs.

Men and women alike find it difficult to judge women or girls by their performance without being distracted by their appearance. The Wiener Philharmonic orchestra only succeeded in hiring female musicians after they started auditioning behind a curtain with shoes off. These elaborate measures were needed to prevent their looks and gender from influencing judgments of their musical performance.

Ann Hopkins, a successful attorney who attracted large clients for her firm, was rated "unfit" for partnership because of her make-up and dress style. She later won a landmark employment discrimination case. Serena Williams won the Roland Garros Grand Slam contest less than a year after giving birth to her daughter. But in the media, disapproval of her black catsuit prevailed over praise of her fitness or athletic achievement.

Women are sad because we know that culturally, our worth stems from our looks. We know this, because if famous, powerful, successful women are primarily judged by their looks, we must be too. We are praised and applauded for being pretty, meanwhile, our blood, sweat, and tears go largely unnoticed. Our accomplishments falter beneath, "She's smart, she's just not very pretty," or are overshadowed by "She did X and Y but isn't she pretty?"

No wonder the confidence of girls and women is chronically lower than that of men and boys. Men and boys are not unilaterally judged based on their looks. Most men, and many women, don't understand this, and so punish and blame women for our lack of confidence.

This is the patriarchy at work. By telling women and girls that our appearances grant us value, the patriarchy systemically usurps the autonomy, intelligence, and successes of women and girls. In doing so, the patriarchy also teaches men to judge women and girls by their looks, creating a reward feedback loop that can look something like this: a woman dresses up, she is complimented by both men and women for her looks, she learns that it is good to look pretty. She takes pains to look pretty, all or most of the time, because she has learned that taking the time to look pretty is more important than taking time to do nearly anything else.

Women are sad because our beauty grants us a privilege that is undeserved and therefore baffling. There is an entire field dedicated to the advantages of beauty: pulchronomics, or the study of the economics of physical attractiveness. Being pretty makes finding a job easier. It makes us more popular in real life, and online. It helps us advance in our careers. Other people are nicer to us. And most insidiously, pretty people earn more money, across all industries, than the rest of the workforce.

The privilege of prettiness dies, though, the moment we are deemed too old, too wrinkled, or too soft to be attractive anymore. We collectively make fun of older women who have had lots of Botox or cosmetic work done, but when you grow up learning that how you look is what gives you value, you are terrified to lose it because then you don't matter anymore.

I was both beautiful and sad because, in navigating the world of dating, I was running head first into an uncomfortable reality. I was learning that being called "pretty" or "hot" or "attractive" doesn't feel good when I have so much more to offer. I was also learning how icky compliments can feel when they drip from the mouths of people I was not trying to look pretty for. In some ways, I was subliminally realizing that one day, my attractiveness would not be enough, and that realization left me feeling listless and more than a little bit angry.

"Attractive women often don't think they're attractive," Dr. T tells me. "They can appreciate the beauty of other women, but for some reason, they can't seem to see any beauty in themselves."

BAD DATES

Nearly a year after I ended my engagement, I went on a date with a trumpet player. We met on Hinge, and judging from his profile, playing the trumpet was his job, his hobby, his side gig, his wife, and his mistress. Our conversation was light and fun, and I was pleased with how intelligent he seemed. It only takes a few weeks of half-hearted "how was your day?" and "hey," texts to lower the conversational bar. My friends warned me to set my expectations low when I met men on dating apps, so that I could avoid inevitable disappointment. I was new to dating apps and navigating the world of online dating felt like a part time job. The day before we were set to meet in person, he texted me: *I'm so excited to meet you!* and I felt the same way. He was fun and flirty via text, and I drove an hour to Long Beach to meet him. When we met in person, he pulled me into a sweaty, half-embrace, his forehead shimmering with moisture, his hands cold and clammy. I was relieved that he looked like his pictures, for the most part, but as we walked to a nearby bar, my light infatuation quickly dwindled. He was braggadocious and self-absorbed. He called his ex-girlfriend, "crazy" and "unmotivated," and talked about how he had "saved her" by allowing her to live with him while she went to school. He talked endlessly about his trumpet, and when we sat down at the bar, he waved his finger at the bartender and called her "darling."

We drank old fashioneds made with Maker's Mark, luxardo cherries floating in our glasses like tiny Christmas ornaments. I fidgeted in my chair and watched him talk, staring too long at his mouth. His teeth looked too big, and he had a weird habit of licking them. After we left the restaurant, chatting and tipsy, I asked him, "What are you looking for?"

He kissed my hand, and said, "A good time." If I hadn't been tipsy, I might have left right then, but I didn't.

After finishing our drinks and biting our cherries, we went back to his place to walk his dog around a small, manmade lake. Someone was fishing, and I remember thinking how funny it was, to fish in a manmade lake that was more of a pond, in a city park in one of the largest cities in Southern California. Even in a concrete jungle, we all crave nature. After we circumnavigated the lake, he invited me inside. I stood on the sidewalk outside of his apartment and looked at him doubtfully, saying, "I better go home."

"Just for a minute," he prodded.

The alcohol made my brain feel soft and pliable, and I found myself agreeing. I missed having a partner, and craved the intimacy I had with Chad; the easy companionship of making dinner together every night, binging shows on Netflix, or listening to podcasts together during long road trips. We sat on his couch, and I listened to him talk more about trumpets and orchestras and students and nothing. I was wearing a romper, and his clammy hands found their way up my bare thighs. Eventually, his mouth found mine. It had been so long since I had been held or kissed, and my body wanted intimacy, but I didn't want it with *him*. I barely knew him, and I didn't even *like* him.

Nevertheless, I didn't say no when he pulled out a condom. I didn't say no when he entered my body. My body wasn't saying no either, but my brain knew it was bad—not the intimacy necessarily, but the intimacy with *him*, in this way, on this night, when I didn't feel heard or understood. I knew I could have said no, *should* have said no, but (and this is a big but), I was scared. Not that he would hurt me physically, but that I would be met with anger or indignation or shame. My desire for intimacy and approval was so deep that I disregarded all my needs to please him, and I didn't even *know* him.

After the sex was over, we cuddled for a few minutes, my hair splayed across his chest, his low voice droning on and on. How asinine. I lingered for a few moments before throwing on my clothes. "Thanks," I mumbled, not looking at him.

"I'll call you," he called out, still lounging in bed.

I cried as I drove home, a rare, Southern California rainstorm spotting my windshield. I never saw him again, pressing the decline button when he called the next week.

As a young adult, I was taught that sex was bad, and that abstinence was not only what God wanted from me, but the only sure way to prevent a pregnancy. My discomfort around sex and my body stretched far into adulthood, and the side effect of never learning about sex, relationships, or communication was awkwardness followed by shame. As I drove home in the rain, I promised myself to withhold physical intimacy until mental and emotional intimacy had been established. Boundaries around our bodies are important, but I was never explicitly taught that, and I was never taught how to set them. I wondered how many men and women, boys and girls, are just like I was—walking around with soft, squishy boundaries and allowing input from other people to determine their thoughts and actions, putting the happiness and comfort of others ahead of their own happiness, or even safety.

***

I took a long break from dating, and more than a year after I met the trumpet player, I went on a date with a marine, another man I met on Hinge. He called me one morning before we met, after I gave him my number.

"Hello?" I answered, confused and a bit disoriented as it was only 6 in the morning.

"Sarah!" he nearly yelled into his phone. I could tell he was driving and figured that was why he was shouting. It turns out that he was just a loud talker.

"Good morning!" he bellowed, "I thought I'd call so I could hear your voice."

"Well… hi," I answered, rubbing my eyes.

"Did I wake you?" he screamed, scaring my inner ear drum.

I switched the audio to speaker and turned the volume all the way down.

"Just got up," I answered. "Are you…on your way to work?"

"Sure am!" He said, "I've just really enjoyed our text conversation and wanted to hear your voice."

I felt myself soften, my initial disdain for his early morning call giving way to some sort of flattery. *Wow*, I thought, *he must really like me.*

Or maybe he was inconsiderate, but I didn't know that yet.

A few days later, I found myself at a restaurant overlooking the ocean in Dana Point. I drove my motorcycle, insisting that he not pick me up.

The moment our eyes met when I entered the restaurant, my heart sank. He looked nothing like his profile photo and as we embraced for a quick hug, I found myself at eye level. There is nothing wrong with a short man, and there was nothing wrong with him. However, I felt duped and misled, and as he scarfed down his overpriced burger, my annoyance gave way to disgust. Not for who he was, but for *how* he was. Plus, it was obvious that we simply wanted different things. He didn't like to stay in one place too long, he described himself as, "not the type to put down roots." By now, I was ready for a real relationship. I wanted to find someone who could build a life with me, and he was nothing I was looking for. It seemed obvious to me that continuing the night would be a waste of each other's time.

When the waitress brought the check, I insisted on splitting the bill, 50/50.

"I'm a gentleman!" he exclaimed, slipping his credit card into the waitress's hand and flicking my card back across the table to me.

I caught my card, eyeing him warily. I didn't want him to think I owed him anything for buying me dinner. I snapped a rubber hair band that was around my right wrist, a nervous tick I picked up during my time in therapy.

"Thank you," I said, snapping the hair band again. I glanced down at my wrist and the pink splotches I'd made. This small physical discomfort calmed me, and I made light small talk as we exited the restaurant.

He walked me to my motorcycle, which was parked a good distance away from the restaurant in a mostly empty parking lot. The harbor in Dana Point was notoriously sleepy, catering to the retired crowd so everything closed early.

"I had a good time," he said smiling. I wondered if he *had* had a good time, or if he was simply oblivious to the fact that I hadn't.

"Thank you, really," I said, trying to avoid lying.

"I hope I can see you again," he said, wrapping one arm around my shoulders.

I caught my breath as he pulled me closer, his head leaning in as my head tipped backwards.

"What," he said, startled, "you don't want to kiss me!?"

"No, I don't." I answered quickly, cold sweat coating my underarms, "I'm sorry, I just *don't*."

I glanced around the parking lot, hoping we weren't alone.

"Did you just want a free meal?!" he said, "God, I'm so sick of this!" It was dark, and we stood beneath a lone streetlight that illuminated our unfortunate predicament.

I took a step toward my bike. "That's not it at all, and you should know that," I said, "really, it was lovely to meet you."

I put my key in my bike's ignition, letting the engine warm up a bit. He was still standing there, staring at me, one of his hands slack while the other curled into a fist before uncurling again. I was nervous now. I glanced around and spotted a couple cutting through the parking lot on their way to the harbor. I caught the woman's eye and held her gaze.

"I'm *so sick* of this!" my date said, almost yelling.

I inadvertently shivered, quickly buttoning my jacket and pulling out my riding gloves. When I glanced up, I saw the couple walking toward us, the woman waving cheerfully, as if she knew me.

"Hi hun!" she exclaimed, walking up to me and pulling me into a big bear hug. "How've you been?" She looked at me hard for just a moment, before turning toward my date. "And who are you?" she asked.

The marine seemed deflated. "Danny," he mumbled, "nice to meet you." He looked at me, "I better be getting home," he said, "early morning,"

"Take care," I said quietly, and he rushed away.

I waited until he was across the parking lot and climbing into his pickup truck before turning toward the couple, my eyes widening in astonishment. "How did you know?" I asked, but didn't let them answer before blurting out, "*Thank you.* Thank you so much, he was getting so angry, and it was only our first date, and I didn't say anything I just didn't want to kiss him and I never thought, I *really* never thought he would do anything but you never know and—"

"It's okay," the woman interrupted me. "I could just tell something weird was happening and I know what it's like to be in a bad situation. This is my husband Jake, and I'm Jen."

I hugged her again and shook Jake's hand. "Nice motorcycle you've got there," he said, which I appreciated simply because it was *not* a nice motorcycle. It was a 2003 Kawasaki Concours, a touring sports bike that went fast, but was really annoying to take care of because I constantly had to clean the carburetor.

I giggled a bit at the absurdity of his compliment. "Thank you," I said, "I started riding last summer during the pandemic, it's really fun but this," I said, gesturing down at my motorcycle, "is not a nice bike."

He grinned, and Jen laughed. "I'm trying to be nice!" he exclaimed.

"I'm Sarah, by the way."

"Well Sarah it's lovely to meet you and I hope you get home safe," Jen said.

"We're going to watch you leave," Jake stated. "Drive safe, okay?"

"Always," I promised. I got on my bike, wiping condensation from the visor of my helmet. "Thank you," I said again. "Really." I felt like I should say something more, but I didn't know what.

As I drove home, my anxiety about the date melted into gratitude for Jen and Jake and pride in myself for standing my ground. When I arrived back home, I checked my phone and had a dozen messages from the marine, all ugly and hateful. I blocked his number and climbed into bed with my cat. I was nearly done reading *Wild* by Cheryl Strayed, and underlined a quote from Mary Oliver. *Tell me, what do you plan to do with this one wild and precious life?*

MIKE MIKE

More than a year later, I attended a Friendsgiving party hosted by my friend Andrea, who was the kind of friend born of transience and convenience. We met shortly after I moved to Southern California through Bumble BFF. I was looking for friends because I had just moved. Andrea was looking for friends because she had lost all of hers. She was wild and self-obsessed, always looking for the next conspiracy theory to explain life's mysteries. She once paid hundreds of dollars to have an exorcism and claimed that it not only healed her injured wrist, but that it gave her the "gift of discernment." After her revelation, she wore a "Jesus is my Savior and Trump is my president" T-shirt that stretched over her pregnant belly. Andrea and I aren't friends anymore, but if I hadn't known her, I would have never met Mike Mike.

Andrea lived in a 150 square foot apartment that was only accessible through a back alleyway, in the same apartment building where Mike lived. Her Friendsgiving party was necessarily held outside in the courtyard of the apartment where fifteen or so people gathered. Mike let Andrea use his oven to cook a turkey, as her apartment did not contain an oven, a kitchen sink, or a kitchen.

I was fresh out of a weird, three-month relationship with an awkward 20-something boy man, who would have been sweet if he hadn't been so stifling. I was also being pursued by a different man who I had worked with once, and who had recently gotten divorced and temporarily moved into a communal living building in San Francisco. He called me a few days before Friendsgiving to tell me about his plan to travel around the world, before asking me to "give him a chance."

"I just want to take care of you," he said, which was nice and all, but he didn't have the capacity to take care of anyone but himself. I worked with him in that we worked for the same organization. However, he was in Northern California, and I was down south with all the finance bros and surfers and intolerably beautiful women. Because I was feeling a bit avoidant and a bit grossed out, his display of unrequited affection made my skin crawl.

There was also a guy I'd met on Bumble, who found out I'd booked a trip to the Copper Canyon in Mexico to have an "immersive cultural experience" and run a marathon. He signed up too, then kissed me with hairy lips under a sweaty, star-soaked Mexican sky and promptly stopped communicating a few weeks later.

As I walked up to the apartment complex for Friendsgiving, I was feeling profoundly fatigued by the male species. Maybe I'd date women for a while, I thought, or move to a new city, or travel to Iceland and dunk my head into one of their crystal-clear lakes to remedy whatever it was that was causing me to be perennially single.

Mike was sitting in a lawn chair in a flannel jacket and gray stocking cap. We started chatting, and I discovered that he'd once worked in sales but now worked in fundraising. I once worked in fundraising but recently accepted a job in sales. "We should connect on LinkedIn," I said, hoping he might have a connection to an employer who offered an above average salary and cheap healthcare.

He chuckled and said, "Sure, let's connect on LinkedIn." And we did.

Later that night, I learned that Mike had just turned 53. I was 28, and because of our age difference, I didn't consider him a likely prospect. Mike didn't showcase any of the same hesitation and offered me a shot of his finest whiskey before spinning me around the courtyard as music blared from a portable speaker. My friends looked on with raised eyebrows before disappearing into Andrea's hovel to change into swanky dresses. After the dishes were cleared away and the courtyard restored to its previous state, we all walked downtown to a bar called Marine Room. Mike leaned against the bar and ordered me an old fashioned, and I admired how easily he carried himself, yet how unassuming he was. Mike was nothing like the egotistical finance bros I was used to meeting. He wasn't excessive or hiding insecurity beneath a veil of cockiness. He just *was*, and I instinctively felt like I could trust him.

Later, we walked outside, the cool salt air snapping at our skin. "Can I kiss you?" he asked, ever the gentleman. "Of course," I answered, letting my earlier hesitations fade into a soft hum. So, beneath a single streetlight, backed up against the cold brick of an upscale bar, we made out until our lips were numb.

After dipping back into the bar for an hour or so, Mike walked me back to where my car was parked outside the apartment building. "You can sleep on my couch," he offered, "if you're uncomfortable driving home."

I *was* uncomfortable driving home, but I was also in a new era, or so I told myself. My new era was one in which I did not go home with a man on day (or night) one, even if that man was utterly sexy and safe all at once. I raised my eyebrows at him. "I'm not that easy!" I exclaimed, the whiskey buzzing warmly in my veins. I was determined to drive the few miles home, even though I knew better. In my mind, it felt safer to drive home than to sleep on Mike's couch.

"At least let me know when you've made it home," he said, and that's how he conveniently tricked me into giving him my phone number.

Weeks later, Mike went home to New York for the holidays, and I went home to Wisconsin. Every night, I'd lay in my parents' guestroom and talk to Mike for hours, my voice low as my parents slept a few doors down.

"I can't wait to see you again," he'd say, and I'd smile wide, wondering if he could hear it.

That was more than three years ago, and although we're no longer together, Mike steadfastly remains one of the best men I've ever known. He patiently waited while I slowly but surely lowered my guard. He listened intently and supported me wholeheartedly. I didn't know that a safe, secure, healthy love was possible. Mike Mike showed me that there are men who are safe, and trustworthy, and for that, I will forever be grateful.

IRRITATING FUDGE

"Sarah!" my mother chirps warmly over the phone one dark December evening. I hear my father grunt before rumbling, "I'm here too, ya know."

"How are things," my mother asks, and I hear dishes banging. She's probably loading the dishwasher, and I wonder what they had for dinner. Today feels like a meatloaf night, or maybe a frozen pizza, or maybe she went ahead and made her own, dough and sauce and all.

"I hate people," I say, and my father immediately perks up. "Oh, people are the worst," he says. "Loud, stinking, annoying people."

"On my flight home from New Jersey," I say, launching into a diatribe before anyone can sideline the conversation, "I sat next to some guy who took his shoes off *and* his socks." I repeat, "His socks! Can you believe it??"

"Oh jeezus," my father moans. "You'll never convince me to get in one of those hell tubes! Flying, metal godawful tubes, they pack you in there like sardines. You'll never get me on one of those things."

This is the reason I called, to have my father validate my hatred of people with his own, much greater, hatred of people. I live in a city, but my father lives on 120 acres. His ability to avoid the general public is something I profoundly envy, especially when I'm trapped in a metal hell tube.

"It's not just that," I continue, "the flight was delayed so we sat on the runway for a full hour before going anywhere."

"Say it ain't so!" my father crows, laughing as my mother sighs heavily into her receiver. They still have a home phone number, so they can each have their own receiver, so long as one is not dead or lost or otherwise compromised.

"Well, how was the trip *generally*?" my mother asks, attempting to avert the conversation away from all this griping and complaining, to no avail.

"Stupid," I say, "I was only there for like two days, and we just had all the same meetings we always have." I pause to take a drink of carbonated water, which I inconveniently choke on.

"And I like everyone I work with, but I am getting awfully sick of the numbers. It's all about the *numbers* you know, all we talk about every month is the number and if we'll hit the number and how to reach the number and what to do if we're short of our number and then when the month turns over, the cycle starts again and we're back to zero and talking about hitting the damned *numbers*." My work in sales is necessarily numbers-driven; each month, a new quota. Each quarter, new forecasting. Each year, a discussion about how to hit our numbers next year. It's a fun challenge, if at times exhausting.

My father chuckles and grunts, "Big man's gotta get paid," and I'm not quite sure what he means.

"Anyway," I say, filling a gap of silence, "what did you have for dinner?"

"Leftover pizza," my mother replies just a little smugly, "homemade."

My mother is the kind of person who takes great pride in making food from scratch. She buys baking supplies in bulk, and spices by the baggie. She meticulously recycles and turns up her nose, ever so slightly, at the offer of a store bought biscuit or pre-packaged cookie. Her philosophy is: if it isn't delicious, I'm not going to eat it. The older I get, the more I admire her pickiness when it comes to good food.

"I could make this better at home," she'll say over a plate of roasted Applebee's chicken. And of course she could, but that isn't quite the point. The point is not having to cook the chicken, and my father, God bless him, is not the type of husband to make dinner.

"What do you want for dinner tonight?" my mother will say in the morning as my father reads the paper with a strong cup of Hills Bros coffee and a plate of buttered toast.

He will grunt and say, "Dunno."

My mother will suggest something entirely reasonable like pork chops or a pot roast.

"Uuuggghh," my father will reply with a look of utter disdain. Sometimes, my mother will make casserole instead, but sometimes she'll go ahead and make the pork chops, my father's griping be damned.

It's fun to complain, especially with someone like him, who is so very good at it. We can go back and forth for hours, like we did after my parent's recent road trip up to Michigan

"There was so much *fudge*," my father said. "It was everywhere! I told your mother, I told her, who needs so much fudge?! Fudge isn't something you eat every day. And on every other street corner, I swear Sarah, there was another fudge shop."

"Well did you get any?" I asked blandly, playing solitaire on my phone while lying in bed. I could tell they were in the same room, on different receivers, their voices echoing between two phones.

"Oh, hell no," he said, taken aback. "I think we got some chocolate covered peanuts, didn't we DD?"

"Yes, and they were very good," my mother said politely, and I presume she thought they were no better than chocolate covered nuts she could have made herself.

"You know where there's *really* a lot of fudge?" my father asks. "Mackinac Island! I told your brother about all this fudge up there and he says I haven't seen anything until I've gone to Mackinac Island. That poor bastard. Pretty funny though, 'you haven't seen anything,' he says, 'until you've gone to Mackinac Island!'"

I've won a game of solitaire by now and have given into full bellied laughter. "Who *does* need that much fudge?!" I nearly scream, my eyes tearing up and my face turning red.

I laughed so much that I forgot why I'd started, but if you really think about it, fudge is preposterous and not that good.

"Fudge is just something you don't need that *much* of," my father is saying. "My god, you need about a knuckle's worth and even that'll make you sick."

Months later, I attended a trade show and found myself talking to a pot-bellied man who was walking around the floor nibbling on a veritable hunk of fudge. I thought about my father, about the "knuckles worth" of fudge, and wondered how much of this hunk this man planned on eating. He offered me a taste, but I'm not stupid. My parents always warned me against taking candy from strange men.

"My God," my father says. "It's really a shame, I liked Michigan, but I just can't. Get past. The fudge." I pictured him gesturing with his hands, emphasizing his dramatic pauses for greater effect. I dissolved into laughter and by now, even my mother was chuckling.

Life is too short to be taken so seriously, so after we hung up our phones, I shipped a single piece of fudge to my father, straight from Mackinac Island.

WHITE CHRISTMAS

"You need to get the *hell* outta California," my uncle tells me.

He's joking, but he's not. We're standing in my grandparents' small kitchen, in a single story, white-sided home in rural Northwestern Wisconsin. Their house is crowded this Christmas Eve, with aunts and uncles and cousins piled onto the small loveseat, spilling over into the dining room, hands dipping into the bowls of nuts and plates of crackers and cheese my grandmother always lays out before Christmas dinner. The dinner *before* dinner, my father likes to say. My uncle, in his mid-50's, has a large white beard and an even larger round belly. If he weren't so grouchy, he could pass for a dressed-down Santa Clause.

"Too many goddamned taxes," he says gruffly. "I thought Minnesota was bad, but we've got nothin' on California."

I don't know what to say to this, so I just point outside, at the heavy piles of drifted snow and say, "Yeah, but we don't have to deal with any of *this*."

He laughs, "What, are you going soft now? Can't handle a little snow? Tell me," he pauses, taking a long drink from his third can of soda, "whaddathey got ya payin' in rent?"

This is a valid question, considering that, at the time, I lived in a 250 square foot studio with a sagging shower floor and a miniature oven that leaked propane. I slept with all my windows open.

"Sixteen hundred dollars," I say, "but I live in a studio. A little one."

At this, my uncle guffaws, pink splotches covering his cheeks, making him look even more like a Redneck version of Santa. "That's criminal!" he says, and my father, who has traveled over from the television to the table full of crackers and cheese, hears this last bit about rent and is compelled to chime in, "I agree! You gotta get out of there," and he pats my back hard, like you might pat a horse if you'd like that horse to gallop now, please.

My brother, who is seventeen months older than me and the complete opposite in terms of temperament, has lived in a two-bedroom, one bathroom apartment in the town we grew up in. There isn't much to do, but the rent is dirt cheap, only $600 a month. His girlfriend moved in recently, so they've been splitting it.

"You could move back here and save a ton of money!" he says, his only contribution to any conversation thus far in the evening. My brother has always been tight with his money, which has resulted in him doing quite well with his fiances. I once visited him when he was living alone, and his cupboards were mostly bare. He was trying to eat everything he had before going to the grocery store, he explained.

"*Everything*?" I asked, eyeing a single can of Bush's baked beans in an otherwise empty cupboard.

It doesn't really make sense, my desire to live near the coast. I spend most of my free time running in the mountain ranges that border Los Angeles and Orange County. I don't swim or do any of the other asinine things people do in that shark-infested, deadly cesspool they call the Pacific Ocean. I tell myself I don't go in the ocean because it's "overrated," but really, I'm just a god-awful swimmer and very scared.

My studio apartment is 1,000 miles away from my family and the cost of living is so high that a six-figure salary barely qualifies me for a standard, no-frills one-bedroom. In my quest to save money, I downgraded my living standard to a studio apartment with street parking, shared laundry, noisy neighbors, and a resident skunk who lives in the garden outside my front door.

One of my neighbors sells drugs, and when I first learned this, I was terrified that I'd moved into an unsafe neighborhood. After a few months, I stopped locking my door and couldn't help but respect his hustle. Besides, he mostly sells weed and mushroom chocolates, none of that hard stuff they're always talking about on the news. Not that I watch the news, but my mother does.

"Did you see," my mother says, "that California is in a deficit? After two years of enormous surplus no less." She pops a chocolate covered pretzel in her mouth, looking satisfied.

"Oh golly, the government always wants more *money*?! Take my money!" my father says, raising his hands to heaven. "What do I need it for anyway?"

"The problem is," my mother says, "that none of these politicians can ever agree on anything. If they could just meet somewhere in the middle—"

"Well, we know that'll never happen," my uncle interrupts, sitting himself down on a cushioned bar stool that my grandmother has strategically placed near the kitchen island for her very fat cat named Wilson. She often calls my brother Wilson by mistake, and although his name is Nathan, the mistake somehow makes perfect sense. A foot stool sits near the bar stool, so the cat can hop from one to the other to reach his final destination, the kitchen counter. On days that are not Christmas Eve, my grandmother fills a plastic syringe with water and blasts cold water down Wilson's throat. He *can* drink water by himself, he simply *prefers* my grandmother's help.

My uncle has unknowingly sat on the cat's bar stool, and Wilson, in his 24 pounds of feline glory, glares up at my uncle angrily before retreating to the Christmas Tree, where he gnaws on a few plastic ribbons that he will later throw up.

The conversation has turned back to the reason we're all gathered. "Play some Christmas carols for us, Nathan," my grandmother all but yells, her hands deep in the refrigerator. My aunt is methodically slicing a pineapple, and potatoes are boiling over on the stove. The kitchen windows are gathering condensation from the heat of cooking and too many warm bodies.

"If you're going to sing carols, I'm going outside," my father announces like a petulant toddler. Within seconds, he slips on his shiny black and red dart ball jacket from the year his team won the state championship, kicks on his thick boots, and disappears into the cold night air, snow sparkling around him like blue-white glitter. His breath makes small clouds, and he lets out a heavy sigh of relief.

My brother decides he'd rather appease my grandmother than protest her wishes, especially on Christmas. He sits down at the shiny wooden piano, cracks his knuckles, and busts out "God Rest Ye Merry Gentlemen." He's never taken a formal piano lesson, just taught himself by ear. I'm convinced my brother received all the genius genetics, and I was left to fend for myself with my abject hyperactivity and an average IQ score. My aunt and mother bust out lyrics intermittently: *God rest ye merry gentlemen let nothing you dismay.*

By the time we've all sat down to dinner, we're half full from snacking and out of easy conversation, so talk turns back to California, the cost of living, and what the hell I'm doing living there, instead of here, in this harsh, frozen winter-scape.

I need to communicate in a way my family can understand, so I don't tell them about the beaches or the miles of wild mountainside or even the fair labor laws and easy access to healthcare. I just say, "It feels like a second home," because the Northern darkness has always felt familiar, but it's the people sitting around this long wooden table that make me feel at home.

IN THE SHORT TERM

Later that same Christmas week, I give my grandfather a hug, his shoulders thin and drooping. He was never a large man, but age and illness have shrunken him even further. At 5'4" I stand taller than him, and at 150 pounds, I outweigh him by a couple dozen. I am strong and sturdy, and my grandfather feels like the maple leaves in late October: dried out and thin, with just a bit of color left in his cheeks. Nothing makes life seem greyer than watching someone transform from a strong, capable man into a shadow.

I thought about the summers I spent with my grandparents, how my grandfather built stone walls with nothing but his strong, sinewy arms and had a garage full of tools and trinkets. He could fix anything. The men in my family are all fixers, and they have ruined me. I had to learn the hard way that not all men can rewire the electrical circuits in a barn or fix a washing machine or change a tire. Not all men can see what is broken and fix it. Most men can't even see that they're broken themselves.

I have never been able to piece together items or understand how things work, in that tear-it-apart-just-to-put-it-back-together way that some people have. My grandfather is one of those people, as are my father and brother. I have spent my entire life trying to understand people, trying to understand myself, and trying to make language mean something. I have failed more times than not because language is an infuriating, absurd thing. But as I type these pages, I can't help but feel like I've told nearly all the stories that I could possibly tell. My grandfather has told nearly none, not because he doesn't have any, but because he was never one for talking. His language was all in his hands, and it wasn't until he started losing his memory that he started talking about his distant past in fits and spurts and circles.

Most of my memories of my grandfather place him outside, stacking stones to build a retaining wall, carrying tuna fish sandwiches outside on a tray so we could eat lunch on a picnic table in a garden, driving his John Deere through the yard and into the woods, shoveling snow, his glasses fogging up when he came inside. My grandfather was a quiet man, and the deep mystery of him has lived in tandem with his steady, reassuring presence. To be seen, heard, and known is such a profound relief and I wonder if or when my grandfather ever felt it. Most of all, I wonder who made him feel that way, and how.

People say a lot of things about dementia; it's caused by this food or that chemical or could be prevented by this supplement or that exercise routine. As it stands, there is no cure and my grandfather's forgetfulness comes in slow, undulating waves. My grandmother reminds him who one of his granddaughters is. How she had a baby months ago, and the baby's name. Family is a tangled, messy thing, a shoebox full of lost and found items that have everything to do with one another, or nothing. I have family members I wouldn't recognize if they stared me in the face, and I wonder if that's how my grandfather feels now that his short-term memory is all but gone. Her name sounds familiar, but he can't quite place her. That face, so much like his own, but who is she?

He is in a nursing facility now, where certified nursing assistants use a machine to lift him onto the toilet, or out of his wheelchair and into bed. Most people with dementia have good days and bad days, and some days, my grandfather can play a few rounds of 500 rummy until he starts forgetting the rules or playing the wrong cards. Some days, my mother goes to visit him and stays for an hour, and he doesn't recall her being there at all.

When I visited over Christmas, my whole family went to the nursing home, myself and my parents, my grandmother, my aunts, and cousins. My brother brought his wife and their nine-month-old baby—a great-grandfather and his great-grandson, so far apart in the circle of life that the end has nearly met the beginning. One rose-cheeked baby sitting on the lap of a ninety-year-old man, both smiling and happily oblivious.

As I sat with my grandfather, I looked around the room, past the fish tank and a stack of books, past the cheerful Christmas tree to where a handful of people sat alone. One woman sang to herself, and another attempted to shush her. They talked about what was on the dinner menu and gazed outside where icy wind whipped across a frozen, snowless landscape.

"We have to bring Sarah to the airport," my mother was saying, "she has to go back home today."

"Where's home?" my grandfather said, looking up at me through his thick glasses.

My heart broke a little bit as I answered, "I live in California now."

He nodded, as if to say, "yes, right," as if he's annoyed at himself for forgetting. Some days, he doesn't understand that he can't go back home, that this nursing facility is where he will spend the rest of his days. I wish I could slip inside his brain for a while and reappear with a better understanding of him and his story. For now, I content myself with holding his hand for a moment, wishing that this fleeting moment in time could stretch on forever.

SEASONALLY DEPRESSIVE

It was Easter Sunday over two and a half decades ago, and I was nearly beside myself with excitement. I found my Easter basket that morning, full of candies and toys. It was in the oven, and it took me an eternity to find. My brother's basket was in the dryer, and he was already halfway through his Easter candy by the time I found mine.

My grandmother hosted a big Easter gathering each year. She and my grandfather would hide dozens of easter eggs and give us kids a list of eggs to find: 4 small yellow eggs, 2 large purple eggs, 4 small pink eggs, etc.

This Easter, however, the house wasn't just full of pastel decorations and jellybeans. There was an argument happening, and I struggled to discern what it was about.

"Christians play *games*, Denise!" my grandmother was yelling at my mother.

"I just don't think it's a good idea," my mother protested, "it has nothing to do with being Christian," and I understood that I needed to be quiet and contained. Mom and grandma were having a fight, and if I made it worse, I worried I wouldn't be able to search for eggs later. I tried to tune out the argument, but my grandmother's house was small. The kitchen bled into the living room, and I couldn't go outside without drawing attention to myself. Their fight began escalating, and I felt a knot of anxiety grip my throat.

"That's it! I'm leaving!!" I heard my mom exclaim, her voice an octave lower than normal. I peeked around the corner of the kitchen to see my mother zipping her long brown jacket. She shimmied out of red slippers and into a pair of snow boots, then flung open the door and marched out into the April chill. There were a few crocuses peeking through a thin layer of spring snow. It was not new that my mother and grandmother were fighting.

They fought all the time, and I always felt compelled to fix things. Sometimes I'd make myself useful by setting the table or clearing away dishes. Sometimes I'd try to distract everyone with a funny joke or antic. And sometimes, I'd simply flee because running away was just easier.

Eventually I figured out that the reason for their argument was, like most arguments, grounded in idiosyncratic morals and worldviews. My grandmother thought it would be fun to hide a $100 bill in an easter egg. Whoever found it would get to keep it. My mother saw the potential for one or many of us kids to throw a fit or cause some other unnecessary drama. From the perspective of an adult, I find myself agreeing with my mother. As kids, we were obsessed with fairness and nothing about a single, crisp $100 bill would have seemed fair.

My father has been caught in the middle of these arguments since they married, siding first with his wife, then his mother, then removing himself entirely and hiding out in the garage until things have blown over. My mother will complain about my grandmother, and my grandmother will complain about my mother, and the mother-in-law/daughter-in-law feud that is a tale as old as time will reign strong.

From my perspective, my mother was and still is the strongest, most beautiful woman I know. My grandmother was and still is a source of comfort and compassion. When two of your favorite people are at odds, it's hard to pick sides. "I just don't know what to do sometimes," I tell a new therapist now, as a 30-year-old adult with lingering issues. I started seeing her in the dead of winter, shortly after daylight savings, when the entire world seemed so bleak and so disturbingly sad. I'm seeing this therapist over Zoom, and she sits close to the screen so all I can see is the top half of her face. "They've just never gotten along, and I always felt like I had to smooth things over. It was exhausting," I tell her forehead.

We're talking about my family because my therapist asked about my family. Are my parents still married, do I have any siblings, what other extended family was I close with, etc.

"Do you feel like the physical distance between you and the rest of your family is a useful buffer?" she asks, "I mean, you can sort of just get off the phone if things are getting out of control."

"Things don't get out of *control*," I say, immediately annoyed and defensive. Plus, has this woman ever talked to her family on the phone? It's pretty hard to hang up on your mother or grandmother without a damn good reason. "Besides, it doesn't bother me very much *now*, I'm saying it really affected me as a kid."

"When kids act as intermediaries, they often become anxious," she says, and I notice her writing something down. I roll my eyes internally and wish I could lean through the computer screen to see what she wrote.

"Maybe I am more anxious than not," I admit, pausing briefly to edit my statement, "I mean I'm definitely more anxious than not."

The therapist sits back, so her entire face is visible for the first time since we started the session. She smiles. "It's good to have that understanding of yourself," she says. "Now tell me," she continues, "what was it specifically that inspired you to reach out to me?"

I don't answer, because I'm not quite sure what to say. I'm not sure it's possible to find the right words to describe a feeling as wide and murky and mysterious as the ocean. Depression can feel like that: an ocean, and I was in the middle of one with no idea how to find the shore.

I tried all the normal things that Google suggested to help with a bit of seasonal depression: talk to a friend, go for a walk, rest, go for a run, make something with your hands, take a bath, touch grass, look at yourself in the mirror and say something entirely asinine like, "you're pretty today," or "at least your feet don't stink," or "you have both kind and youthful energy," or "dogs really seem to like you."

The holiday season is always, and for no reason that's obvious to me, the season of sadness. Some years, it swallows me whole and spits me out in late March, blinking and blinded. I don't know which way is up and if someone told me to turn left at the next stop sign, I'd probably stare blankly. Amid this depression, I long earnestly for an escape. I want to hear what it sounds like when strangers sing in their cars. I want to scream underwater. I want to hug all the people who break promises and ask them why.

Sometimes there is no reason for feeling down or depressed. It comes in waves and half of my brain knows it will lift while the other half wonders what it feels like to die. And then I get anxious. And then I think about empty churches and empty movie theaters and get sad all over again.

I tell my therapist how my cat needs medication for his hyperactive thyroid. I tell her about a hurricane that was supposed to hit Southern CA but petered out into a bland rainstorm. I tell her about how I just ran through Joshua Tree, the rising sun like a jellyfish glowing on the Eastern skyline. I tell her how much I love the desert, how I'm not sure why. Maybe because it seems so empty, while so full of life.

After our session, I sit next to Mike on our blue-gray couch. He stares at his phone, and I stare at my feet and think about where they'll take me next. Maybe I'll run up the coast, as far as I can. Maybe I'll run every street in this sleepy beachside city. Probably I'll go back to the mountains, where I first nursed a broken heart and learned how to be strong again.

I pick at a scab on my forearm from where I recently burned myself on a hot frying pan. I wonder if it's wrong to sort of like how it feels, not the picking but the burning. I wonder if I should burn myself again, not by accident, or if anyone would notice.

HOME AGAIN

I'm home visiting the farm in mid-August, when the sweet corn is perfectly ripe and the sun still stretches its long, sherbet fingers into nighttime. It's been nearly seven months since my last visit, and I'm startled by how deeply the landscape has changed. My mother is showing me the vegetable garden. "Looks like I need to pick beans again," she mutters, and squats to the ground, her hands deep in a green bean plant. My parents started planting beans on a fence years ago, so the plants grow from the ground up, higher than my head. I start plucking the ripe beans, too, eating one for every three I toss in the bucket at my mother's feet.

My father walks by and says, "Getting back to your roots, eh?" pronouncing "roots" like "ruts."

I smile, because it feels so satisfying to have my feet in the dirt of their vegetable garden, and I'm not sure they'll ever know how good it is, even now, to come home.

Some people think that if you've seen one small town in America, you've seen them all. I fear that might be true; my hometown might be like all the other small towns scattered across the country, just with a different cast of characters. Mr. Wilson, the old gym teacher, is now the librarian. The daughter of our high school basketball coach went away to college, got married, and settled down across the street from her parents. Now, she has two little girls of her own and has taken over the head coaching job. Voting day takes place at the municipal building downtown, which also houses the damp, musky library full of outdated books and large, clunky computers. My hometown still publishes a local paper once a week, a two-to-four-page bulletin detailing town news, high school sports, traffic tickets, and classified ads.

I scan this week's paper at the Formica-topped kitchen table as my mother washes lettuce in the kitchen sink. It was front-page news that the municipal building, which is on a list of historic structures, has been approved for a federal restoration grant.

New carpet, updated pipes, things like that. It was also front-page news that the school district lost some funding, so is now in a budget shortfall. A large sum of the overall deficit was made up by the school sending out notices to all the families who still owed lunch money for the previous school year. Some families owed hundreds. Some owed over $1,000. It is the plight of rural America to live with less, and to be proud of it. Maybe even to be hungry, but not admit it. Or maybe, to put off paying one bill, like lunch money, in favor of paying a more pressing expense, like the mortgage or the heating bill.

Because I left home a long time ago, just after I turned 18, I've started romanticizing rural life. *Wouldn't it be marvelous to live off-grid?* I think, as I sit in heavy traffic. *Wouldn't it be nice to grow and hunt my own food?* As I overpay for organic eggs and peppers that are hopefully not coated in pesticides. *Wouldn't it be nice to live somewhere quiet?* I say to Mike, as we eat dinner together while our upstairs neighbor practices Irish dance in the unit above us. *Wouldn't it be nice to take a full, deep breath of the pure, clean air?* I think, as I stand on a mountaintop overlooking the smog that shrouds Los Angeles.

And yes, all of that might be nice, but I know that it's nic*er* in my imagination, just as the lure of Hollywood is better in our collective unconscious than it will ever be in modern life. For all my romanticizing, I am reminded that rural life is considerably less convenient than life in other places. My parents have a septic system that needs pumping, a propane tank that needs refilling, well water that needs to be periodically tested, and trash that needs to be sorted and hauled to the dump. They have a lot of space, but a lot of space requires a lot of maintenance. They spend countless hours mowing the lawn, removing snow, cleaning up after thunderstorms, and tending to their gardens. There is no convenience store within walking distance and going anywhere requires more than a little bit of driving, and my hometown isn't even as remote as many rural towns. There is a Walmart a twenty-minute drive away, grocery stores, and a small state university. As I help my mother pluck beans, I am reminded that in rural America, there are always chores to be done, and the sun never seems to be awake quite long enough.

My brother bought a house down the street from the high school we both attended. My parents and I make the short drive to his house one evening, and I drink up the views of the town slowly rolling by, the library and gas stations and small Chevrolet dealership. The bars and antique shops, the winding creek that dumps into the dark and swirling St. Croix River. I used to stare at the town on the bus ride to school, growing weary of the same landscape that flashed by day after endless school day. Now, my tiny hometown stands in sharp and welcoming contrast to the views I've grown accustomed to living in Southern California: the endless blue Pacific, narrow beaches full of tidepools and coves, the infuriating traffic snaking up Pacific Coast Highway or jammed together on the five. Traffic is the one thing everyone has in common here. We have all been stuck in hours-long slowdowns, bumper to bumper and honking our horns and gazing miserably through streaky windshields. Traffic is a great equalizer, like death. It doesn't matter how rich or poor you are, how handsome or how homely, how motivated or depressed, how intelligent or how stupid. We have all sat miserably in traffic and it is nearly impossible to avoid. Driving through my hometown, I smile at the few stray cars moseying down the main thoroughfare. *There is plenty of parking here*, I think, *and so much space.*

My grandmother likes to tease me that I've become a "city person." City people say "dinner" instead of "supper." City people don't like dirt under their fingernails or bug bites on their ankles or hard physical work. City people are unimpressed by the natural beauty that exists outside the bounds of their concrete jungles. City people think it's fun to pick beans once, without any thought of planting, watering, weeding, or canning them. Of course, my grandmother has not spent very much time in any large city, and it's almost impossible to truly understand a place you haven't lived in or loved.

Being unimpressed with otherness is not new or unique to rural America in general or my family in particular. Later that evening, I laugh as my father recalls his trip to the Grand Canyon, "Just a big hole in the ground," he grunts. Similarly, he grumbles about the drive to Minneapolis, where he and my mother scooped me up from the airport days before. "Couldn't pay me millions of dollars to live in that godforsaken city," he says.

And I believe him. Because if there is one thing my father has taught me, it's that there is no place on earth quite as precious as home.

THE END

On Mike's 55th birthday, we went out to dinner with his cousin Scott, and Scott's longtime girlfriend, Heather. The drinks flowed all afternoon, and our hotel balcony wine morphed into Mai Tais at a high-top table in a restaurant on the ocean side of Pacific Coast Highway called the Royal Hawaiian. Scott works in television and dresses entirely in black. Heather works in fashion and tells me that it's perfectly okay to wear denim on denim. I jab Mike's arm and say, "*See?* Heather *knows*." Earlier that week, Mike and I had a friendly row regarding the wisdom of denim-on-denim. I said yes, but Mike said no. In all fairness to Mike, he didn't really give a damn.

Scott is five years younger than Mike and they act like brothers. They're doing the thing that only men do, which is give each other an enormous amount of shit with the understanding that they don't really mean it (but they do).

I turn toward Heather, who is asking me a question about running, "I'm not sure I understand," she's saying, "why you do these crazy races. What do you get out of it?"

The Mai Tais are hitting me hard, and my brain is pleasantly foggy. "You know," I say slowly, "I just really enjoy them. It's not like I'm making any money from them or anything, but I think," I say, looking up at the copper ceiling, "it's always valuable to do hard things."

The conversation turns back to work and family and vacations and friends. I didn't think about her question for weeks. To be completely honest, I didn't think of a good answer until I was halfway through writing this book.

I spent over a decade in the throes of an eating disorder, trying to make my body run fast while starving it thin. It wasn't until I reached my mid-twenties that I understood what it meant to be healthy. It wasn't until my late twenties that I had the opportunity to combine a healthy body with a healthy mind. I am still running because I still haven't reached my full potential. It's enormously simple and surprisingly profound: I don't want to stop in the middle, and the metaphor extends far beyond running. For so long, I didn't have the strength to live a full life.

I want to say yes to every new experience, opportunity, or challenge life offers, and racing is just a fractional part of that. Her question gave me pause at the time, but now it almost seems beside the point. In a moment of nostalgic longing, I wish I could go back to the Royal Hawaiian and edit my answer. I suppose in a way, I have.

ABOUT THE AUTHOR

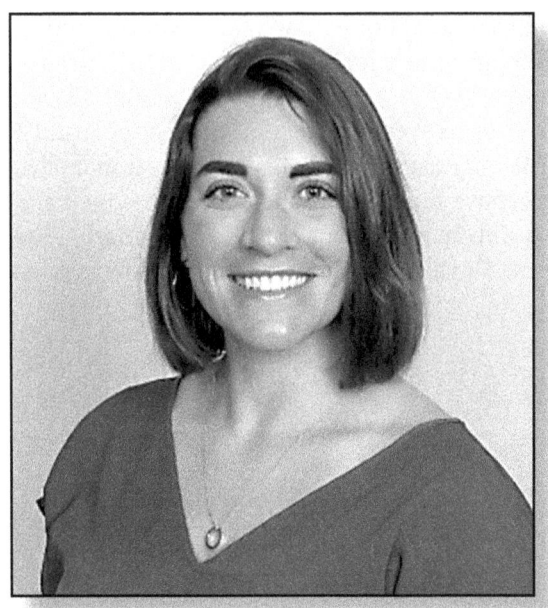

Sarah McMahon is a poet & ultra runner based out of Costa Mesa, CA. Originally from a tiny town in Northwestern WI, her work draws upon her experiences growing up in rural America. She studied English at Bradley University under the tutelage of Illinois poet laureate Kevin Stein, earning a B.S. and M.A. in English. In 2023, she self-published a book of poems called *Dirt Girl*, and has been published in *Hamilton Stone*, *City Works*, and other presses.

ACKNOWLEDGEMENTS

Enormous thanks to Eric Morago and the team at Moon Tide Press for believing in my work and my vision. This book would not have been possible without the editing expertise of Katrina Prow, who skillfully and gently kept my narrative on course. Nor would the cover art convey my story so well without the thoughtful design of Andrea Smith.

I would be remiss to not thank the many teachers who nurtured my love for writing and storytelling, from grade school all the way through my Master's degree, most especially Mrs. Suckow, Mrs. Myers, Dr. Stein, and the late Dr. Brill de Ramirez.

Thank you also, to the many medical professionals who helped me through and out of my eating disorder, especially Dr. T. and Amy the Dietician.

Thank you to the Southern CA writing community for validating my voice and existing as a safe and supportive place for art to thrive. Similarly, I owe the Southern CA ultrarunning community a debt of gratitude for helping me believe in myself.

Endless thanks to my family for your constant, unconditional love.

And finally, thank you to Mike for your enduring kindness and for reading every single one of my poems.

Also Available from Moon Tide Press

The Elephant of Surprise, Charles Harper Webb (2026)
Outliving Michael, Steven Reigns (2025)
Prayers with a Side of Cash, Kathleen Florence (2025)
Somewhere, a Playground, Rich Ferguson (2025)
The Tautology of Water, Giovanni Boskovich (2025)
Take Care, Mark Danowsky (2025)
Dilapitatia, Kelly Gray (2025)
Reluctant Prophets, J.D. Isip (2025)
Enormous Blue Umbrella, Donna Hilbert (2025)
Sky Leaning Toward Winter, Terri Niccum (2024)
Living the Sundown: A Caregiving Memoir, G. Murray Thomas (2024)
Figure Study, Kathryn de Lancellotti (2024)
Suffer for This: Love, Sex, Marriage, & Rock 'N' Roll, Victor D. Infante (2024)
What Blooms in the Dark, Emily J. Mundy (2024)
Fable, Bryn Wickerd (2024)
Diamond Bars 2, David A. Romero (2024)
Safe Handling, Rebecca Evans (2024)
More Jerkumstances: New & Selected Poems, Barbara Eknoian (2024)
Dissection Day, Ally McGregor (2023)
He's a Color Until He's Not, Christian Hanz Lozada (2023)
The Language of Fractions, Nicelle Davis (2023)
Paradise Anonymous, Oriana Ivy (2023)
Now You Are a Missing Person, Susan Hayden (2023)
Maze Mouth, Brian Sonia-Wallace (2023)
Tangled by Blood, Rebecca Evans (2023)
Another Way of Loving Death, Jeremy Ra (2023)
Kissing the Wound, J.D. Isip (2023)
Feed It to the River, Terhi K. Cherry (2022)
Beat Not Beat: An Anthology of California Poets Screwing on the Beat and Post-Beat Tradition (2022)
When There Are Nine: Poems Celebrating the Life and Achievements of Ruth Bader Ginsburg (2022)
The Knife Thrower's Daughter, Terri Niccum (2022)
2 Revere Place, Aruni Wijesinghe (2022)
Here Go the Knives, Kelsey Bryan-Zwick (2022)

Trumpets in the Sky, Jerry Garcia (2022)
Threnody, Donna Hilbert (2022)
A Burning Lake of Paper Suns, Ellen Webre (2021)
Instructions for an Animal Body, Kelly Gray (2021)
Head *V* Heart: New & Selected Poems, Rob Sturma (2021)
Sh!t Men Say to Me: A Poetry Anthology in Response to Toxic Masculinity (2021)
Flower Grand First, Gustavo Hernandez (2021)
Everything is Radiant Between the Hates, Rich Ferguson (2020)
When the Pain Starts: Poetry as Sequential Art, Alan Passman (2020)
This Place Could Be Haunted If I Didn't Believe in Love, Lincoln McElwee (2020)
Impossible Thirst, Kathryn de Lancellotti (2020)
Lullabies for End Times, Jennifer Bradpiece (2020)
Crabgrass World, Robin Axworthy (2020)
Contortionist Tongue, Dania Ayah Alkhouli (2020)
The only thing that makes sense is to grow, Scott Ferry (2020)
Dead Letter Box, Terri Niccum (2019)
Tea and Subtitles: Selected Poems 1999-2019, Michael Miller (2019)
At the Table of the Unknown, Alexandra Umlas (2019)
The Book of Rabbits, Vince Trimboli (2019)
Everything I Write Is a Love Song to the World, David McIntire (2019)
Letters to the Leader, HanaLena Fennel (2019)
Darwin's Garden, Lee Rossi (2019)
Dark Ink: A Poetry Anthology Inspired by Horror (2018)
Drop and Dazzle, Peggy Dobreer (2018)
Junkie Wife, Alexis Rhone Fancher (2018)
The Moon, My Lover, My Mother, & the Dog, Daniel McGinn (2018)
Lullaby of Teeth: An Anthology of Southern California Poetry (2017)
Angels in Seven, Michael Miller (2016)
A Likely Story, Robbi Nester (2014)
Embers on the Stairs, Ruth Bavetta (2014)
The Green of Sunset, John Brantingham (2013)
The Savagery of Bone, Timothy Matthew Perez (2013)
The Silence of Doorways, Sharon Venezio (2013)

Cosmos: An Anthology of Southern California Poetry (2012)
Straws and Shadows, Irena Praitis (2012)
In the Lake of Your Bones, Peggy Dobreer (2012)
I Was Building Up to Something, Susan Davis (2011)
Hopeless Cases, Michael Kramer (2011)
One World, Gail Newman (2011)
What We Ache For, Eric Morago (2010)
Now and Then, Lee Mallory (2009)
Pop Art: An Anthology of Southern California Poetry (2009)
In the Heaven of Never Before, Carine Topal (2008)
A Wild Region, Kate Buckley (2008)
Carving in Bone: An Anthology of Orange County Poetry (2007)
Kindness from a Dark God, Ben Trigg (2007)
A Thin Strand of Lights, Ricki Mandeville (2006)
Sleepyhead Assassins, Mindy Nettifee (2006)
Tide Pools: An Anthology of Orange County Poetry (2006)
Lost American Nights: Lyrics & Poems, Michael Ubaldini (2006)

Patrons

Moon Tide Press would like to thank the following people for their support in helping publish the finest poetry from the Southern California region. To sign up as a patron, visit www.moontidepress.com or send an email to publisher@moontidepress.com.

Anonymous
Robin Axworthy
Conner Brenner
Nicole Connolly
Bill Cushing
Susan Davis
Kristen Baum DeBeasi
Peggy Dobreer
Kate Gale
Dennis Gowans
Alexis Rhone Fancher
HanaLena Fennel
Half Off Books & Brad T. Cox
Donna Hilbert
Jim & Vicky Hoggatt
Michael Kramer
Ron Koertge & Bianca Richards
Gary Jacobelly
Ray & Christi Lacoste

Jeffery Lewis
Zachary & Tammy Locklin
Lincoln McElwee
David McIntire
José Enrique Medina
Michael Miller & Rachanee Srisavasdi
Michelle & Robert Miller
Ronny & Richard Morago
Terri Niccum
Andrew November
Jeremy Ra
Luke & Mia Salazar
Jennifer Smith
Roger Sponder
Andrew Turner
Rex Wilder
Mariano Zaro
Wes Bryan Zwick

www.ingramcontent.com/pod-product-compliance
Lightning Source LLC
Chambersburg PA
CBHW031320160426
43196CB00007B/598